"The authors tease out a radical vision of an embodied yoga where the body is no longer 'just a body' but a 'tool' of discovery. In its most fundamental expression, the body in yoga *reveals* mind. The achievement of their approach is that, through a newly framed yoga, they accept the paradox of the body, which is that it can stand mute as a stone, and yet say something wholly other."

**Joseph Rubenstein**, *professor emeritus of anthropology and ritual at Stockton University*

"This is the book that yoga desperately needs as it struggles to evolve effectively in the modern context. It offers critical academic and practical insight and covers a wide range of topics of central concern to serious practitioners. Do not expect a pious re-appraisal of the tradition of yoga here. This book contains radically new thought on what yoga could mean for us now."

**Adam Keen**, *founder of Keen on Yoga, an online community and podcast platform, and international yoga teacher*

"This book is a challenge that's well worth the effort. The writing is stimulating. It's radiant with brilliant flashes of intelligence and insight that elevate our understanding of yoga. It's a harbinger that shines a light on the emerging transformative power of yoga in the West."

**Richard Rosen**, *yoga teacher and author*

"Clark and Greene offer an invigorating and original set of essays, this time directed toward serious yoga practitioners. The authors highlight the complexity and richness that has developed through the past century of engagement between the philosophical and embodied understandings of yoga in India and their evolving global practices."

**Sarah Strauss**, *professor of anthropology and author of* Positioning Yoga

# YOGA AND THE BODY

*Yoga and the Body: The Future of Modern Yoga in the Studio and Beyond* imagines the prospects for physical yoga practice. The authors, writing as advanced practitioners and teachers, share their enthusiasm for yoga and lay out the ways its physical practices can evolve and make an impact upon our understanding of consciousness.

The chapters examine techniques, trends, and beliefs about contemporary practices and then speculate about where these could lead. Topics include the central importance of the body in spiritual experience, the role of emotions and imagination in consciousness, the insights gained through aesthetic philosophy about the nature of reality, and yogic techniques used for exploring the mind, body, and spirit.

This book is for anyone who has ever taken a yoga class and wondered if they are missing something. It is a thoughtful and entertaining guide to embodied exploration for those who are genuinely curious about modern yoga and its future.

**Edward Clark** is the creator and artistic director of Tripsichore Yoga Theatre in London. He is internationally recognised as a teacher of advanced yoga technique and philosophy.

**Laurie A. Greene**, PhD, is a professor of anthropology at Stockton University and owner of Yoga Nine studios. She is the co-author of *Teaching Contemporary Yoga* with Edward Clark.

# YOGA AND THE BODY

## THE FUTURE OF MODERN YOGA IN THE STUDIO AND BEYOND

**Edward Clark**
**Laurie A. Greene**

Routledge
Taylor & Francis Group
NEW YORK AND LONDON

Designed cover image: Cover photo by Jean-Philippe Woodland

First published 2025
by Routledge
605 Third Avenue, New York, NY 10158

and by Routledge
4 Park Square, Milton Park, Abingdon, Oxon, OX14 4RN

*Routledge is an imprint of the Taylor & Francis Group, an informa business*



ISBN: 9781032731056 (hbk)
ISBN: 9781032731032 (pbk)
ISBN: 9781003471752 (ebk)

DOI: 10.4324/9781003471752

Typeset in New Baskerville
by Apex CoVantage, LLC

# Contents

# Acknowledgements

The imagery associated with contemporary yoga is largely comprised of exceedingly healthy looking young people in form fitting clothing. We ruefully laugh that there was a time when aging yogis were revered. As longtime practitioners and teachers, we are so grateful to those who have helped us in writing this book of essays because their investment of time and effort in turn gave us the enthusiasm to plough on through with saying what we think needs to be said at this point in yoga's history. We are particularly appreciative of those who read early drafts of one or more of these chapters and offered comments and suggestions. Joseph Alter, Joe Rubenstein, Richard Rosen, Jamal Jones, Sarah Strauss, Adam Keen, and Glen McDonnall – we thank you for your extraordinary kindness. Reading work that is unfinished is difficult and time consuming and offers little reward in exchange. Know that your contributions are in these chapters and have much improved them.

We would also like to acknowledge Anna Moore and the editorial staff at Taylor and Francis/Routledge for their willingness to take a chance on this book well before it was completed. A huge thank you to the amazing photographer Jean-Philippe Woodland for the photograph on the book's cover. A second thank you to Jamal Jones who is always happy to answer vexing questions about Sanskrit language and language history. We also recognise that this is the second time you have gladly offered us your vast expertise on the subject during the writing process.

Inspiration comes from many places and often arises when and where you least expect it. The chapters in this book arose from a variety of everyday insights and experiences. Thank you to David Byrne for his unique and hopeful view of the world as told through his play *American*

*Utopia.* Also, thanks to John Lydon for his compelling delivery of the lyric *Anger is an Energy.* To Kevin Chai, Allegra Chong, Zoe Bloom, Sergio Ruiz, Jorge Garcia, Lady Blue, Lucía Hernández, thank you and *muchas gracias* for entertaining conversations about this material and your dedication to experimenting with these ideas in your own practice and teaching. Finally, thank you to our students who provided a lion's share of the material for the chapter "What Really Matters" and who have helped us thresh out these ideas from the perspective of dedicated practitioners.

# Glossary of Sanskrit Terms in IAST Transcription

| Common usage | IAST | Contemporary Gloss |
|---|---|---|
| Ama | *āma* | 'toxin' |
| Anahata | *anāhata* | 'heart chakra/unstruck' |
| Anjali mudra | *añjali mudrā* | 'prayer hands' |
| Asana | *āsana* | 'posture/stable seat' |
| Ashram | *āśrama* | 'ashram/monastery' |
| Avidya | *avidyā* | 'inability to see/ ignorance' |
| Baba | *bābā* | 'novice yogi' |
| Bhaghavad Gita | *Bhagavad Gītā* | 'Bhagavad Gita' |
| Bhakti | *bhaktī* | 'devotional (practice)' |
| Bhastrika | *bhastrikā* | 'bellows breath' |
| Bhavana | *bhāvana* | 'temple/imagination' |
| Bhramari | *bhrāmarī* | 'bee breath' |
| Bija | *bīja* | 'seed' |
| Brahman | *brahman* | 'eternal reality' |
| Buddhi | *buddhi* | 'discerning mind' |
| Chabutra | *chabutra* | 'raised platform' |
| Chakras | *cakras* | 'chakras/energy vortices' |
| Chaturanga dandasana | *caturaṅga daṇḍāsana* | 'reverse push-up pose' |
| Dharana | *dhāraṇā* | 'focussed concentration' |
| Dharanas | *dhāranās* | 'kinds of concentration' |
| Dharanis | *dharanīs* | 'incantations' |
| Dharma | *dhārma* | 'calling/purpose' |
| Dhyana | *dhyāna* | 'meditation' |
| Drishti | *dṛṣṭi* | 'focus' |

| | | |
|---|---|---|
| Eka grata | *ekā gratā* | 'single pointed focus' |
| Granthis | *granthis* | 'energetic knots' |
| Guru | *guru* | 'enlightened teacher' |
| Guruji | *guruji* | 'enlightened teacher' -hon |
| Hamsa | *hamsā* | 'sacred hand/hand of god' |
| Hatha yoga | *haṭha yoga* | 'physical yoga method' |
| Hatha Yoga Pradipika | *Haṭha Yoga Pradīpikā* | 'important tantric text' |
| Ida | *idā* | 'female energy channel' |
| Ishvara pranidhana | *īśvara praṇidhānā* | 'surrender to the divine' |
| Jogapradipika | *Jogapradipika* | 'hatha yoga text' |
| Kali yuga | *kali yuga* | 'era of darkness/ignorance' |
| Kapalabhati | *kapālabhāti* | 'skull shining breath' |
| Karma | *kārma* | 'action/work/deed' |
| Kirtan | *kīrtan* | 'devotional chanting/ music' |
| Kulā-Arṇava-Tantra | *Kulā-Arṃava-Tantra* | 'tantric text' |
| Kundalini | *kundalinī* | 'female energy' |
| Maha | *maha* | 'great' |
| Maha mudra | *mahā mudrā* | 'great seal pose' |
| Maithuna | *maithuna* | 'tantric priestess' |
| Mala | *mālā* | 'prayer beads' |
| Mantra | *māntra* | 'sacred chanting' |
| Maya | *māyā* | 'illusion' |
| Moshka | *mokṣa* | 'liberation' |
| Mudra | *mudrā* | 'energy seals' |
| Mukti | *mukti* | 'liberation' |
| Mula | *mūla* | 'source/root/foundation' |
| Namaste | *nāmāste* | 'I bow to you' |
| Nadis | *nādīs* | 'energy channels' |
| Nidra | *nidrā* | 'sleep' |
| Ohm/aum | *Oṃ* | 'the sound of creation' |
| Padmasana | *padmāsana* | 'lotus posture' |
| Parsvottasna | *pārśvottānāsana* | 'side angle posture' |
| Parvati | *Pārvatī* | 'Pavarti-Shiva's wife' |
| Pingala | *piṅgāla* | 'male energy channel/ right' |
| Pradipika | *pradīpikā* | 'light/clarity' |
| Prakriti | *prakṛti* | 'evolving reality' |
| Prana | *prāṇa* | 'energy/life force' |
| Pranamayakosha | *prānamayakośa* | 'food (energy) body' |
| Pranayama | *prānāyāma* | 'breathwork/energy work' |
| Pratayahara | *pratyāhāra* | 'sense withdrawal' |
| purashcarana | *puraścaraṇa* | 'preliminary rites' |

| | | |
|---|---|---|
| Purusha | *puruṣa* | 'pure consciousness' |
| Raja | *rājā* | 'kingly' |
| Raja yoga | *rājā yoga* | 'yoga of kings/classical yoga' |
| Rishi | *rishi* | 'sages' |
| Samadhi | *sāmadhi* | 'total absorption' |
| Samasthiti | *samasthitiḥ* | 'equal standing' |
| Samkhya | *Sāṃkhya* | 'nondual philosophy' |
| Samsara | *saṃsāra* | 'cycle of rebirth' |
| Samskara | *saṃskāra* | 'mental impressions' |
| Sannyasin | *saṃnyāsin* | 'renunciate' |
| Sarvangasana | *Sarvāṅgāsana* | 'shoulder stand pose' |
| Siddhis | *siddhis* | 'super powers of enlightened' |
| Shakti | *śakti* | 'shiva's mate/female energy' |
| Shala | *śālā* | 'studio/school' |
| Shavasana | *śavāsana* | 'corpse pose' |
| Shisya | *śiṣya* | 'student/devotee' |
| Shiva | *śiva* | 'shakti's mate/male energy' |
| Shive Samhita | *Śiva Saṃhitā* | 'tantric text' |
| Shushumna | *suṣumnā* | 'central energy channel' |
| So hum | *so'ham* | 'I am that chant' |
| Sutras | *sūtras* | 'strings/aphorisms' |
| Swami Vivekananda | *Svāmi Vivekānanda* | 'modern yoga sage' |
| Tadasana | *tādāsana* | 'mountain pose' |
| Tapas | *tāpas* | 'ritual heat' |
| Tattva | *tattva* | 'elements of reality' |
| trikonasana | *trikoṇāsana* | 'triangle pose' |
| Ujjayi | *ujjayi* | 'victorious breath' |
| Vasana | *vāsanā* | 'mental impressions/habits' |
| Vayu | *vāyu* | 'wind/energetic movement' |
| Vibhuti Pada | *Vibhūti Pāda* | '3rd chapter of Yoga Sutras' |
| Vikalpa | *vikalpa* | 'imagination' |
| Vinyasa | *vinyāsa* | 'moving physical practice' |
| Vipassana | *vipaśyanā* | 'style of meditation' |
| Vishnu | *Viṣṇu* | 'deity Vishnu' |
| Vratyas | *vrātyas* | 'outcast' |
| Yantra | *yantra* | 'mandala/meditative image' |
| Yoga Kurunṭa | *Yoga Kuruṇṭa* | 'Yoga Kurunta' |
| Yoga nidra | *yoga nidrā* | 'yogic sleep' |
| Yogashala | *yogaśālā* | 'yoga studio/practice space' |
| Yoga Sutras of Patanjali | *Yoga Sūtras of Patāñjali* | 'Yoga Sutras of Patanjali' |

# Introduction

## THE STATE OF MODERN YOGA

There is a significant amount of academic writing about yoga – its history, philosophy, and critiques of the neoliberal aspects of contemporary practice – but there is a surprising lack of formal analysis about the experience of yoga practice itself. Without a body one cannot engage with external reality *or* the internal realm of thought and spirit. By focusing on the experiences of practitioners, and the theoretical implications of these experiences, the body is revealed to be fundamental to both our physical *and* spiritual existence. *Yoga and the Body: The Future of Modern Yoga in the Studio and Beyond* looks at many facets of physical practice that have been left unexamined. These chapters explain the body's importance in the elusive pursuit of the transcendent and imagine how to creatively approach yoga through embodied exploration.

Yoga is a malleable canon of techniques and contemporary yoga does what modern practitioners want it to do – address issues that are relevant to their modern lives. The ancients had different concerns and used yoga in different ways. For example, contemporary practitioners value 'community' as an important aspect of yoga practice, while the ancients used its techniques to engage in solitary contemplation. Similarly, today yoga is viewed as a way to live life to the fullest, whereas, in ancient times, yoga was employed in the hopes of overcoming life's illusions by rejecting an ongoing cycle of eternal recurrence (achieving 'death') through a disregard for the body.

Today, the philosophic value of physical practice, and the premises on which it is founded, are often ignored or dismissed. Physical practice is

DOI: 10.4324/9781003471752-1

typically seen as preparation for more serious meditative or intellectual pursuits – it is understood as a way to live a healthy life, affording one the opportunity to tackle the real work of transcendence. But self-exploration is physically rooted in both the moving body and the senses and it is through both movement and the sensual that one gains their understanding of reality.

Modern yoga claims to be beneficial in promoting health and well-being. These benefits have been studied by a variety of researchers using clinical methodologies. To establish validity, they often remove yoga practice from its normal context, and subject the experience to controls, limiting the information that is considered relevant. Though this offers legitimacy within the scientific community, it is quite different from the way yoga is usually practised. Conclusions based on *average* responses diminish the importance of the wide range of experience of individual practitioners. What the twice a week devotee experiences is different from someone who dedicates their life to yoga. While most studies focus on the practical implications for health and fitness, yoga has always had ineffable goals. The esoteric aspects of yoga are accessible to all practitioners if given the opportunity and guidance to explore this territory. This book investigates many of the factors that have limited or promoted the exploration of the loftier aims of physical practice. Each chapter concludes with commentary which considers the implications of the analysis presented for the ongoing evolution of practice.

## GENERAL THEMES THROUGHOUT THE VOLUME

### The Phenomenology of Consciousness

When discussing the purposes of yoga, one inevitably grapples with defining what is sought – some understanding of the nature of consciousness. We have been vexed throughout the writing of these pieces by terminology – so many words that only partially convey the full meaning we seek or that have one vernacular meaning and other meanings when used technically. In particular, there are five terms associated with the functions of cognition (the mental action or process of acquiring knowledge and understanding through thought, experience, and the senses) that we have come to use very specifically in these chapters because they assist us in elucidating the more ephemeral yogic endeavours. These terms relate to the way body and mind create and sustain the processes of self; of understanding being – 'meaning', 'interpretation', 'reason', 'rationality', and 'consciousness'.

Since the 1990s, cognitive science has focused on features of human cognition in an attempt to understand the concept of meaning. In the past, the acknowledgement of variability in human understanding and worldview, the questions asked, and theories proposed by researchers centred on the importance of language and culture in the shaping of cognition. They assumed that one needed language to assign and understand significance. But, as philosopher Stephen Asma and psychologist Rami Gabriel contend, "[m]eaning is foundationally a product of embodiment, our relation to the immediate environment, and the emotional cues of social interaction, not abstract correspondence between sign and referent" (Asma and Gabriel 2019). They argue, as these chapters do, that meaning is not limited to the symbolic frame. Meaning is fundamentally tied to somatic activity. This has obvious implications for the importance of somatic practice. After some wrangling, we have come to see meaning as a process – akin to what cognitive scientists, linguists, and anthropologists call "meaning making". At the most fundamental level, meaning is what we make of the sensorimotor interactions which happen when the senses deliver data resulting in the production of feelings. This meaning is the foundational substrata of emotion and thought. The motor reactions that happen – the clenching of the jaw or the racing of the heart – are the postural shifts that accompany, or are the grounds for, emotional expression which result in action. The body's response to stimuli facilitates the creation of meaning – it gives one existential significance.

'Interpretation' is something that happens subsequently at another level of awareness. Here, meaning is explained through contextualisation and narrativised through cultural conventions. Complicated versions of these interpretations may eventually arise to conscious awareness. Asma and Gabriel refer to three "strata of consciousness" involved in meaning making – foundational, secondary, and tertiary levels of cognition. As Asma and Gabriel describe:

> [a]ffective science argues that the lowest layers of mind permeate, infiltrate and animate the higher layers. The evolution of mind is the developmental story of how these layers emerged and acted as feedback loops on each other. Such feedback, however, is not strictly just a brain process, but an embodied, enactive, embedded and sociocultural process.
>
> (Asma and Gabriel 2019)

The first or foundational layer contains meaning that is both essential and evolutionarily adaptive. This meaning is affective and is phenomenologically experienced. From this perspective, meaning, and the cognitive processes that create it, are impossible to understand without considering its embodied foundation. In *The Primacy of Movement*, philosopher Maxine Sheets-Johnson (Sheets-Johnson 2011) similarly proclaims the essential nature of the body in meaning-making and, in her analysis, as the motivator of movement. She describes neuromuscular tension as emotionally laden – a "postural attitude". It is the tonicity needed in the body to ready oneself to express an emotion – a necessary substratum of action and a prerequisite for movement. Affirming the foundational necessity of phenomenal experience, she claims:

> Without the readiness to act in a certain way, without certain corporeal tonicities, a certain feeling would not, and indeed, could not be felt, and a certain action would not, and indeed, could not be taken, since the postural dynamics of the body are what make the feeling and the action possible.
> (Sheets-Johnson 2021, 265)

Asma and Gabriel propose that these affective states (basic and normally below the level of conscious thought) play an important role in survival, create a successful social world for mammals, an information-rich niche for human learning, and a "system for ideational salience". They distinguish seven primary/universal emotions or "foundational affective systems" – fear, lust, care, play, rage, seeking, and panic/grief (after Jaak Panksepp 2010), while others have proposed variations of this taxonomy. As they go on to state of the inherent physicality of consciousness:

> Almost every perception and thought has valence, or is emotionally weighted with some attraction or repulsion quality. Moreover, those feelings, sculpted in the encounter between neuroplasticity and ecological setting, provide the true semantic contours of mind.
> (Asma and Gabriel 2019)

Contrary to the semanticist's categorisation of meaning – be it conceptual, connotative, collective, social, affective, reflected, or thematic – Sheets-Johnson and Asma and Gabriel see emotion as intrinsic to *all* meaning. Building on this somaticised meaning, the secondary layer is where contextualisation occurs. Here, experience stored in memory allows for a heightened and individual interpretation of emotional response. Arachnophobia, for example, is a response to one's past frightening experiences with spiders – of meaning making processed at the secondary layer. Startled by a spider on her wedding day, an arachnophobe (who belongs to a culture where disgruntled ancestors appear as spiders to rebuke their delinquent descendants for taboo behaviours) may heighten her initial fear response, while creating a narrative – at the tertiary layer – in which her grandfather disapproves of her marriage. This may evoke an analogy with the concepts of *saṃskāras* and *vāsānas* found in traditional yoga philosophy. *Saṃskāras* are variously hypothesised by Indian scholars as a sort of "karmic residue" that is part of the unconscious. It is more difficult to distinguish *vāsanās* from *saṃskāras,* but suffice to say, they are both theorised as similar to feelings or emotions – as subconscious or preconscious motivators of behaviour (Bienorius 2004, 5).

The meaning attributed to sensorimotor responses is framed by emotional expressions. When one senses the heat of a predator's breath, they have a different reaction than when they sense the heat of an intimate's breath even though the sensation is the same. An initial fear response (a recoil) may be modified (to pleasure) when the lover is identified, or the context (one's head on a pillow) may prevent the recoil altogether. The language used to narrate one's fear response may also calm the initial reaction if that reaction is deemed socially or culturally inappropriate. Knowing that emotions are both essential and problematic for an understanding of human consciousness, how should the yogi continue to explore the self? In this volume, the chapters "Minding the Body" (Chapter 1), "Anger is an Energy" (Chapter 2), and "The Empathic Dilemma" (Chapter 7) thresh out these issues for the modern practitioner who, unlike the ancients, has access to research findings in physiology, evolutionary biology, neuroscience, and other cognitive sciences.

If 'meaning' and 'interpretation' presented challenges, this was also the case with descriptions of thought itself. Reason and rationality are two processes through which meaning is framed as understanding. 'Rationality' is consistent with scientific reasoning and is independent of our sensory experiences – it is generally "rigid, rarefied, mechanical, and governed by explicit laws" (McGilchrist 2010, Chapter 10, kindle). On its own, therefore, rationality is a poor tool for investigation of the ephemeral where imagination and contingency are ever-present components of direct exploration and experimentation. 'Reason', on the other hand, allows one to attribute meaning absent conclusive or complete information – "it is flexible, resisting fixed formulation, shaped by experience, and involving the whole living being" (McGilchrist 2010, 330). It is based on the strong possibility of some particular situation. It is better suited to the yoga practitioner's interaction with the novel, unknowable, or ineffable nature of theorised universal consciousness. But the use of reason does not mean that the yoga practitioner abandons rational thought. Rationality is utilised in the service of reasonability. One makes use of rational constructs when explicit information, in the form of sensory stimuli, is available to make definitive analyses. One may creatively expand into the realm of reason when their explorations make encounters with the inexplicit difficult to unequivocally interpret. For the practitioner who relies purely on experiences that are explicable through rational thinking, the exploration into consciousness appears improbable, if not impossible.

Finally, we encountered difficulty when defining 'consciousness' itself. From the perspective of yoga philosophy, consciousness is ephemeral yet fundamental. Contemporary practitioners, however, have largely come to believe that consciousness is knowable and embodied. In a modern interpretation of *haṭha* yoga traditions, they seek, through bodily refinement (rather than philosophical pursuit), to achieve a refined mental state (their "true self" or "best self"). In addition to knowability, there is the modern question of whether consciousness is singular or innumerable. Yoga traditions propose that there is a singular 'consciousness' (*puruṣa*) that comprises reality. An individual's consciousness is considered an illusion since it is a transitory material manifestation of the singularity of the immaterial *puruṣa*. Enlightenment is the realisation of this singularity. But the modern practitioner, interacting in the quotidian world, has no choice but to engage with their own consciousness and the consciousness of others. This is particularly salient in the modern practice environment that is, more likely than not, to be a group rather than solitary setting (as was the practice of traditional yogis). The modern yogi plays with, and reacts to, the consciousness of others in their community and the information they can glean from physical interactions with others. Additionally, the rejection of materiality, so commonly accepted in discourse on yoga (even in contemporary circles), denies the centrality of the body in the pursuit of yoga's higher goals. Yet, in traditional *haṭha* yoga texts, it is acknowledged that one cannot engage in the exploration of consciousness without a body (see *Haṭha Yoga Pradīpikā* (1:12) and "Minding the Body", this volume, Chapter 1), and in contemporary practice, to fully manifest the materiality of one's "best self" is a definitive spiritual act. The chapters in this book explore these contradictions and suggest ways in which they may be re-examined.

## Grappling with Self and Other

Some other terms we struggled to represent with clarity and consistency were Other/other and Self/self. 'Self', in its upper-case form, is meant to refer to pure consciousness (*puruṣa*) as the ultimate realisation of nonduality. Early on, we became pleased with a definition of yoga: "Yoga is the study of self and reality and their interactions". This definition is so broad – something like saying it is the study of all existence and it can certainly include various permutations of the meaning of self. The 6th century BCE saw a philosophic preoccupation with locating a primal substance from which all phenomena were derived, and the essence of what any individual might appear to be, was postulated to be this same primal substance – an irreducible self, devoid of any personality and characteristics. This version of self is indistinguishable from the self of anyone else. In fact, it is also indistinguishable from any *thing* because it too, in its irreducible state, has no describable features and is not recognisable through the intellect – though one metaphor often used is "the light of pure consciousness". Whether such a state or experience even exists is debatable, but we refer to it often because so much of yoga practice may have originally been premised on seeking it. We have distinguished this form of consciousness with a capitalisation – 'Self'.

It is difficult to unequivocally state that others' use of self refers to something else – where expression like "true self" or "foundational self" or "best self" are used, its context usually indicates that they are not referring to an indescribable and eternal form of consciousness. So, all of these other "selfs", we indicate with a lower case – 'self'. One place where this distinction became a challenge was where practitioners conflated self-realisation (based in the material experience of the individual self) and Self-realisation (based in the imagining of an ineffable universal Self) as indistinguishable endeavours.

It is equally difficult to know what authors remote in time may have meant by a term like *puruṣa* (pure consciousness). Commentary on it does give perspective – it is something real, but not tangible (in that it cannot be apprehended by the senses). We favour a contemporary rendering of its meaning as being "potential". It is all things that could happen, however remote their contingency, but nothing in it is impossible, nor is much of it likely. The nature of it is distinct from anything in materiality (that which has become). Something that has *become* is already in a process of annihilation; its structure is constantly altering. The nature of potentiality is its possibility, and this possibility is timeless because it is real only in that it could happen, not in its material actuality. Whether a physical yoga practice is likely to unequivocally reveal the primal substructure of reality is debatable as is the answer to whether or not this fundamental structure (or state) is what may have been meant by expressions like "cosmic consciousness", "enlightenment", or *puruṣa*. Potentiality does give modern practitioners a reasonable starting point for investigating spiritual (non-material) matters. It is not material, but it is also not magical.

Another convention that we use is an upper case O in the term 'Other'. We use this to distinguish *everything* that is not the self. When we define yoga as being "the study of self and of reality and their interactions", we are saying that yoga is the study of the 'Totality' (or the 'Absolute'), but that in this study, it is possible to identify as the self and see that it *is* distinct from what is perceived as Other. Arguably, much of yogic pursuit over the centuries has been a striving to eliminate this distinction – the ambition to see all as one. To broach this possibility, it is necessary to acknowledge that there is, for practitioners, such a separation. Upper case Self requires the understanding that self and Other are actually comprised of the same thing. Lower case self and Other present a myriad of possibilities for their expression and interpretation. The yoga practitioner is faced with an intriguing number of ways to interpret themselves and reality. The latitude with which each of us invent reality – the Other – is probably only matched by the breadth of interpretation we make of our self. The Self – if one follows a traditional understanding of *puruṣa* – is not interpretable; indeed, is not possible to even apprehend with *buddhi* (the intellect). The Self (*puruṣa*) is a category of reality that is wholly remote and unknowable by the material world and its workings (including the intellect). We reckon that interpretation is a delightful process. It makes artists of all of us. The only danger is the inherent thought that we have got it completely right – that our version of self and Other is the true one. Not so – as with any artistic project, it hints at the truth or provides but one tantalising perspective.

Because the premise of Self is tenuous, we have looked at where the tendencies in contemporary yoga might profitably lead. Rather than dismissing the body as a vehicle that, at best, is a goad to overcoming itself to find the Self, we consider how the body gives many routes to understanding the self and, possibly, will provide insight into the Self (or hints to its existence or lack thereof). Reality *is* experienced through the body although the idea that the mind and body are separate persists; usually with the mind seen as superior. The mind is thought to sort through the information the body delivers and then makes sense of it. But it may be more pertinent to *think* that the body really is the mind – a process of negotiating the Other.

## DEFINING ĀSANA AND VINYĀSA

In the physical practices of contemporary yoga, there are two major systems – *āsana* and *vinyāsa.* Though many sources are content with defining *āsana* as "stable seat" and *vinyāsa* as "to place in a measured way", these definitions give scant indication of how they are understood and practiced by modern yogis. Each conceives of the Totality (self, reality, and the processes of their interactions) in different ways. In this volume (and elsewhere), we define *āsana* and *vinyāsa* in ways that reflect the realities of modern practice. *Āsana* seeks a version of the self and reality that is foundational and unchanging and rationalises its physical techniques as ways to achieve stillness. *Vinyāsa* considers the nature of reality and self to be something that is consistently undergoing change. Its physical techniques involve sustaining continuous movement. In *āsana,* at its most extreme, there would be only posture with no movement and, in *vinyāsa,* only movement with no posture. As the *āsana* system presumes there to be a changeless and indestructible foundation underpinning self and reality, it does not require the existence of time because duration would mean that things have changed. *Āsana's* pursuit of stillness is meant to prevent the body/mind from engaging with the world – creating through sensual engagement, a persuasive, but perishable, illusion of transient activity. *Vinyāsa* provisionally assumes time to be something that unfolds, or flows, at an even rate – that the rate of change in reality is consistent. The techniques of *vinyāsa* attempt to synchronise with the evenness of the flow of time by pursuing an evenness and synchronisation of breath, movement, and thought – a recognition of the rate of change of the self and reality's being. *Āsana* tries to find an eternally extended moment of undifferentiated consciousness whose prime characteristic is changelessness and *vinyāsa* is trying to perceive a process of continuous flow where there are no moments of stillness, only constant transition. Because *āsana* is always tending toward stillness and *vinyāsa* toward sustained movement, the physical techniques employed are often very different. *Āsana* attempts to place the weight in postures in such a way as to minimise the effort used to sustain the posture in stillness. The parts of the body aim to stack up in alignments that are exquisitely balanced. Movement out of a posture then requires a volitional effort – it does not just happen because of external influences like gravity. *Vinyāsa* places the weight in such a way as to encourage movement so there is an inclination to keep the movement sustained. With each inhale (or exhale), the action commenced at the centre of the body would result in a loss of balance if not altered on the exhale (or inhale) or mitigated by expansive effort away from the centre. These premises are meant to facilitate the way the practitioner approaches the world. The comparative absence of sensual input in *āsana* is meant to lead the practitioner's attention inwards, ultimately divorcing them from both the information of the senses and from inner mental processes. Theoretically, when these are stripped away from the practitioner, the yogi ceases to identify with these transitory processes and comes to recognise they truly reside in a more primal and foundational state. This state is theorised to be the same for all other things in reality – a changeless, indestructible, and eternal place of simple being. So, by stripping away the vestiges of life, the aspirant is meant to find that self and reality are the same. The process of *vinyāsa* is quite the opposite. Here, the practitioner seeks to move their attention outwardly. They actively cultivate sensual appreciation as a way of combining their self with reality. They attempt to recognise that reality is ever influencing change in themselves and they, in turn, are influencing reality. While *āsana* seeks to find a simple state of being that is a bedrock of reality by looking inward, *vinyāsa* seeks to expand the volume of consciousness from a single inner point to include, ultimately, awareness of the whole of reality.

## GRAPPLING WITH SCIENCE

The accumulation of knowledge, much of which is gathered through scientific inquiry, should not be ignored. But as briefly mentioned, we must also take into account the limitations of the scientific method. The problem with a wholly analytic approach to the body, or the objectification of thought, is that it distances one from actual experience. Even the delight of thinking is understood, by some practitioners, to be deceptive or unreal – thoughts stand in the way of an understanding of truth due to their transitory nature. For instance, the early Greek philosophers were fascinated with natural phenomena and found pure delight in conjecture, but, by the time of the Stoics, this thoughtful astonishment was replaced by an intellectual coolness in Eastern and Western philosophy. The primacy of perception became something like "My sensations are merely temporary phenomena of only passing significance". But the exciting thing about sensations is that they are real! Sensing and meaning making are not abstractions – they are the substance of lived reality.

Much of the objectivity found in the analytical approach is accomplished through reductionism – the practice of analysing and describing a complex phenomenon in terms of a single or more fundamental cause, especially when this is said to provide a sufficient explanation. Reductionism is common for a variety of reasons, but mostly it is employed as the result of experimental controls on variables. For example, an experiment looking at the way yoga effects health might isolate and test the efficacy of practicing *ujjayi* breathing on cortisol levels. The isolation of this single variable allows for conclusions to be made that exclude other potential variables that may be responsible for the reduction of stress hormone in isolation or in conjunction with breathing practice. Likewise, reductionism is also at work within the research question from the inception of the experiment, which begins by limiting what is being studied. This research bias is difficult to eliminate and arises from preconceptions about the nature of reality. The assumption here being, "yoga relieves stress", so we should, therefore, figure out what aspect of yoga is responsible for stress relief experimentally. One could just as easily have presumed, "yoga causes stress", and design an experiment to understand this causation – but this is not what we assume to be true. The enemies to experimentation and research are presupposition and assumption, and yet, it is what we must necessarily employ to ask questions and devise experiments. The alternative is to use a multivariate analysis – one that considers a variety of variables and does not control for any of them. Such experiments are virtually impossible to carry out when using quantitative techniques, and risk being exceedingly messy compared to the elegance of controlled testing. In truth though, multivariate qualitative analysis offers greater measures of validity[1], as they simply study a phenomenon in the natural world without the limitations required by the experimental setting.

It is this multivariate experimental perspective that we believe will take yoga into the future. An immersion into the natural setting in which practice occurs with an openness to any sensual information that may arise. If one sees the yoga of the ancients as a perfectly formed system, yoga ceases to be about experimentation – the answers are already known. Modern yoga must be about experimentation if it is to evolve in the future. The assuredness of one's beliefs stands in the way of gaining knowledge and the process of transformation spoken of in Chapter 3, "A Thing of Beauty". The reductionist thinking that arises from this certainty, likewise, stimies both observation and analysis. Scientific knowledge is heavily predicated on numbers – quantitative data. Numbers are perceived as authoritative, and as such, they are seductive, but numerical data is a poor measure of experience, as is discussed more fully in Chapter 8, "Myths and the Negotiation of Reality". Throughout the volume, we acknowledge the authority of the scientific method and its strengths and weaknesses, but emphasise the limitations of quantitative data and methodological controls for understanding the experience of the practitioner.

## MORE QUESTIONS THAN ANSWERS

These chapters are written for serious yoga practitioners. In this volume, we have no intention of definitively describing yoga or answering, once and for all, esoteric questions about the nature of reality let alone how yoga will specifically evolve. What we do hope to do is spur practitioners to ask questions and use their imaginations to look to what yoga can accomplish through its development in the future. We want the reader to be curious about their experiences – to see the great potential in their practice – one which vastly surpasses the everyday goals most popular today – health, fitness, well-being, and self-confidence. To assist in this effort, we include a section at the end of each chapter with our take-aways from the arguments presented. This commentary emerges from our own discussions about the immense potential available in yoga as a practice, and our speculations about where yoga might go and exactly how it might get there.

## BOOK CONTENTS

### Section I: The Experience of Practice

The three chapters in the first section ask how the physical practice of yoga might be used to advance the pursuit of self-realisation – the discovery of the self and its relationship to the Other – in modern times. Restrictions to this advancement are found in the strident beliefs and assumptions made by the discipline in its post-colonial evolution (as a product for Western consumption) and in the reliance on the undisputed sacred knowledge of ancient yogis. The importance of the body is analysed as the site for lived experience, the source of meaning-making, and as a vehicle for change. The physical reality of emotional response is noted as are the experiential and cultural aspects of understanding emotions and their role in motivating action through the attribution of meaning. The value the yoga community gives to emotions is discussed as are the philosophical implications of these attributions – distinguishing between good (desired) and bad (undesirable). The chapters reveal the lack of distinction between the body and the mind and question whether the privileging of the mind still dominates practice today. The related, yet distinct, processes of reason and rationality are used in efforts to understand the ineffable. Both involve imagination, however, only reason allows for interpretation based on context and frees one from the restrictions of thinking within known parameters. Reason allows one to use logic (rationality) to explore beyond what is already known.

### *"Minding the Body" (Chapter 1)*

Across time, space, and culture, human beings have at least one thing in common: they reside in bodies that function in similar ways. This chapter examines how bodily experience provides a substrata of information that is interpreted in the process of meaning making. The body is generally devalued in yoga philosophy as it is believed to be tied to materiality, however, spiritual experience *is* physical. Contrary to Cartesian duality, this chapter suggests that the body/mind is one and the body's kinetic interactions with the Other are the source material for understanding the nature of self and reality. As this chapter demonstrates, the underlying goals and processes of yoga continue to arise from mundane and profound bodily experiences rather than from philosophies found in textual sources or lessons imparted by a *guru.* Absent the body, nothing remains but abstract conceptions. It is through the body/mind that one encounters the spirit; it is not a *conception,* but a lived *experience.* It is only through experiences in the body that one interacts with and creates a version of the world and a version of oneself within it.

### *"Anger is an Energy" (Chapter 2)*

This chapter analyses the role of emotion in yoga practice and its effect on the creation of meaningful experiences and learning. It begins with a definition of emotions and describes the way that "good" or "bad" emotions are viewed and valued differently within the yoga community. Emotions are malleable and mutable and may be either enhanced or dissuaded though contextualisation (experience) and narrativised (culture and imagination). This allows them to be channelled to achieve optimal performance, such as one might experience in the state of 'flow' and is how the potential volatility of a 'reaction' is modified into a focused 'response'. The intensity of emotional response is also considered as are the uses to which it might be put. Ecstasy and rapture are discussed as intense emotional states that are experienced physically and equated with spiritual experience where one sees the true nature of reality.

### *"A Thing of Beauty" (Chapter 3)*

This chapter examines how creativity and imagination can be used in yoga to expand consciousness and lead to the appreciation of the Other. It begins by examining the limits of personality through a discussion of neurobiology. Rigidity of personality is seen as a principal component of social tensions. Aesthetic techniques that may be used to create a less rigid sense of self are considered, along with their capacity to assist individuals in imagining new perspectives and developing empathy for others and their views. The experience of beauty is described as an appreciation of the connection between self and the wider reality and is one method for expanding perception. This expansive appreciation makes it possible to find the extraordinary in the mundane through sensual experience.

## Section II: The Social World

The chapters in the second section explore the core principles of practice in modern yoga and the applications of these principles for modern practitioners. The contemporary cultural realities that privilege concrete and pragmatic ends have led to an apparent shift away from the more lofty and ephemeral aims of traditional practice. The implications of this shift in focus necessarily change the techniques and methods of yogic inquiry and understanding. In particular, yoga has shifted from solitary, individual pursuit of the ephemeral to become a group practice within a studio setting. The triumph of community and style over experienced tutelage and dedication to the *guru* has wrought other changes in yogic ambition – belonging and self-acceptance have gained ascendancy. At the same time, the strong value placed by Western culture on the centrality of the individual has shifted the focus of practice toward personal health and wellbeing. The ascension of these pursuits has come in response to a presumed ever-present toxicity that is seen as a grave threat (that yoga gives its adherents agency to combat) – a reflection, perhaps, of consuming fears about stressors on the planet. Also brought to the fore are the ways that today's 'spiritual entrepreneurs', whether in yoga or aligned fields in the wellness industry, are marketing their wares to consumers. Capitalism (or neoliberalism) begs for novelty, and so, new spiritual products are constantly introduced, sold, and consumed. These chapters grapple with what might allow popularised yoga to regain a more impressive spiritual, physical, and intellectual trajectory and how the knowledge of institutional structures, language, and cultural forces might help us become better consumers of the myriad somaticised spiritual products.

*"What Really Matters" (Chapter 4)*

This chapter argues that Western yoga functions as a ritual of transformation that privileges individual spirit by clarifying and contextualising mundane experience. Through stillness or movement, yoga rituals either strive to negate the body's influence, and thereby the 'self' (*āsana*) or celebrate the body in an active engagement with the 'Other' (*vinyāsa*). Within these emergent ritual experiences, embodied threats to the social order are evoked (e.g., trauma (past), anxiety (future), and toxicity (present)) which may then be expressed in ways that are transformative and cathartic. Yoga practice has transitioned from a solitary enterprise to one that is strengthened by, and legitimised in, intentional communities where these threats are addressed. The role of the traditional *guru* was to obliterate the ego of the disciple; today, however, the teacher is more likely tasked with facilitating their healing – a healing that is both personal and transpersonal, and never completed. Unlike early Western experiments in yoga, modern yoga, in its popularised form, is largely domesticated, making yoga now suitable and accessible to everyone. It is no longer couched within the confines of Eastern religion, but rather in the secular, physical, and spiritual body of the individual practitioner as they seek self-realisation.

*"When Credentialing Doesn't Matter" (Chapter 5)*

This chapter critically assesses the way credentials are making an impact on the development of holistic modalities, including yoga. It asserts that the pursuit of credentials is expanding and their acquisition is used principally as a marketing device rather than for the necessity of increasing knowledge or skill. The phenomenon of the 'spiritual entrepreneur' and their business practices (e.g., the use of multilevel marketing, the assumption of universal suffering, and their alignment with holistic healing modalities) are addressed. The popularity and trust placed in spiritual entrepreneurs is supported through an analysis of the implications of strength of feeling, the placebo effect, and intuition as tools of the profession.

*"Why Language Matters" (Chapter 6)*

The language of yoga serves a number of functions – it expresses the nature of the ideal self and the universe/reality, signals identity to others, and affirms shared values within the yoga community. This chapter looks at the jargon and (often unconscious) ways of speaking in contemporary yoga and how language and language use change as culture changes. In particular, the important and productive role of 'floating signifiers' like 'yogic' and 'the work' and 'the practice' are analysed. The use of Sanskrit, chanting, gesture, voice and affectation, and the vocabulary of positive manifestation and nonjudgement are understood as linguistic conventions for communicating in the yoga community of practice. The chapter points to the need for greater cognisance of the way language is used to limit or encourage meaningful experience.

**Section III: The Transmission of Knowledge**

The chapters in this section explore the processes of creation and transmission of knowledge. The study of the metaphysical is not achieved by the same tools and techniques used in science. The means through which we set out to understand the ineffable are both productive and problematic. Myths and metaphors are necessary tools in the use of one's imagination. They allow us to begin from a place of understanding absent clear demonstrable truths, but they may also stifle our progress if interpreted as literal rather than metaphorical hypotheses. Empathy is useful for exploration of the Other, but it is often an inaccurate tool that may lead to false evaluation or overidentification. Technique is necessary in any somatic practice, but it can inhibit aesthetic discovery if overemphasised. These chapters explore means by which we might move forward to understanding the indemonstrable. Through the application of reason and rationality, a balance of idealism and pragmatism, and through holistic rather than reductionist thinking, we suggest ways to remove roadblocks to understanding the ephemeral.

*"The Empathic Dilemma" (Chapter 7)*

This chapter examines the intrinsic value of empathy and explores the potential uses and abuses of empathic knowledge. It questions the unchecked valorisation of the ability to empathise by focusing on the complexity of empathic understanding and how it may help or hinder the relationship between individuals, particularly in the context of teaching and learning. Empathy is not a quality of a person, but a skill learned through social interaction – it facilitates information gathering. The ability to share empathy makes the reaffirmation of group identity or ritual intensification possible and encourages compliance to group norms. Sensitivity is a function of the nervous system in contrast to empathy. The dilemma when relying on empathy is that, although an experience feels powerful and authentic, it is invented within the self, and so, only purports to be the feeling of another. Despite this dilemma, empathy is presented as a powerful tool to imagine and engage with the Other.

*"Myths and the Negotiation of Reality" (Chapter 8)*

This chapter explores how yoga currently contextualises itself within society and the cosmos through myths and metaphors and suggests how these might meaningfully evolve. Myths and metaphors are used to explain the unknown and underpin a culture's worldview. Traditional myths of yogic origin and nonduality are contrasted with contemporary myths of toxicity and healing, pilgrimage and journey, and words and numbers. In particular, metaphors of light and darkness are explored as powerful elements of traditional and contemporary yogic myth. Finally, the conservatism found in yoga scholarship and practice is compared to reductionist, literalist, and fundamentalist thinking found in other disciplines.

*"The Future of Technique" (Chapter 9)*

This chapter looks at the future of yoga practice techniques and considers the importance of embodiment and whether the body is to be denied or utilised in the process of achieving yogic goals. Yoga has evolved in the West along with a system of institutions and prescribed rules for physical practice. As with all institutions, the yoga industry seeks to establish and maintain power over competing institutions and the people who adhere to their strictures. Developments in future yoga technique are imagined – inspired by other physical disciplines and areas of psychology and philosophy where more research has been completed. This chapter seeks to answer how one strives for enlightenment or other lofty attainments where results can be replicated and subjected to scrutiny. Included in this analysis are propositions for the techniques of *prāṇāyāma*, *prātyāhāra*, *dṛṣṭi*, and the physicality of *āsana* and *vinyāsa* movement.

## IN DEFENCE OF OFFENCE

When writing a book of critical chapters that challenge aspects of an ancient and sanctified practice, one risks offending. For a discipline to evolve – to develop its philosophy and practice – one must ask questions that, to some readers, may appear irreverent. During the Enlightenment, for example, people questioned the sacred knowledge of the church in the name of science. Though we certainly aren't subject to formal charges of heresy, there are still some orthodox practitioners and researchers who will find our questioning offensive. It is not our intention to offend, but to present the discipline of yoga as a dynamic living system with varying practices that change over time as the culture(s) of its practitioners change – rather than a singular practice whose truths were already manifest in full by the ancients. There might be some who say, that as humans of the *kali yuga* (era of ignorance), we have lost much of the wisdom of the ancient sages, or that we are incapable of understanding its profound premises. This may be true, but this reprimand might also be a way now (as it may have also been in the past) to assert the unquestionable authority of certain sages and others who stand to benefit from positions of power and influence. In either case, to bring yoga into a place of analytical inquiry, necessitates what every modern scientific study demands – to question existing premises, subject them to rigorous testing, and possibly arrive at new or amended conclusions based on the results. Therefore, we ask provocative questions and through academic and physical research, experimentation, and analysis, we arrive at potential conclusions that avoid the cognitive dissonance resulting from attempts to marry science with alchemical beliefs of the past.

Some readers of the first manuscript of this book were concerned with our critiques of disreputable practices in the wellness community. These concerns are valid. It is not our intention to lay blame on particular individuals or institutions, but simply to hold a mirror to the realities of this new industry, as one would to any other for-profit enterprise. In addition, we do not see how the discipline of yoga might be improved, or its integrity maintained, without an acknowledgement of these highly visible and often problematic issues. Ignoring these issues will harm yoga and the wellness industry in the eyes of the larger public – especially those who wish to disparage yoga or who dismiss it as trivial.

It seems equally, if not more, offensive that the flaky sidekick on any modern sitcom is likely a yoga teacher or practitioner selling the benefits of manifestation or crystals. She (usually) is attractive and likeable, but not very bright or inquisitive – the subject of side eyes and only tolerated because, well, "she is a *good* person". What a disappointing contrast to the perception of yogis of yore who undoubtedly offended the Hindu establishment with their violation of caste sanctions and taboos as well as their antisocial behaviour, yet who were feared and respected for their ascetic discipline.

The arguments presented in each chapter draw on research from a variety of disciplines, most notably anthropology, art, and psychology. We speculate, but support these speculations, with evidence from contemporary scientific research, our own experience within the community, and with reference to past practice and both ancient and modern philosophy. To this end, we hope that the chapters in this book spur more questions from our readers and also encourage them to engage in their own experimentation and analysis. In this way, the discipline of yoga can become a place where the questioning of authority whether textual, historical, or interpersonal is not only tolerated, but encouraged.

## NOTE

1. Validity refers to how accurately a method measures what it is intended to measure. It produces results that correspond to real properties, characteristics, and variations in the physical or social world.

## REFERENCES

Asma, Stephen and Rami Gabriel. 2019. "United by Feelings". *AEON* 22 August. Accessed 18 December 2023. https://aeon.co/essays/human-culture-and-cognition-evolved-through-the-emotions.

Bienorius, Audrius. 2004. "Play of the Subconscious: On the Saṃskāras and Vāsanās in Classical Yoga Psychology". *Acta Orientalia Vilnensia* 5: 168–184.

McGilchrist, Iain. 2010. *The Master and His Emissary: The Divided Brain and the Making of the Western World.* New Haven: Yale University Press.

Panksepp, Jaak. 2010."Affective Neuroscience of the Emotional BrainMind: Evolutionary Perspectives and Implications for Understanding Depression". *Dialogues in Clinical Neurosciences* 12 (4): 533–545.

Sheets-Johnson, Maxine. 1999. "Emotion and Movement: A Beginning Empirical-Phenomenological Analysis of Their Relationship". *Journal of Consciousness Studies* 6 (11–12): 259–277. Accessed 12 March 2022. https://www.academia.edu/8548014/Emotion_and_Movement.

Sheets-Johnstone, Maxine. 2011. *The Primacy of Movement – Expanded Second Edition (Advances in Consciousness Research).* Amsterdam: John Benjamins Publishing Company.

*The Hatha Yoga Pradipika.* 1997. Translated by Pancham Sinh. 5th edition. New Delhi: Munshiram Manoharlal Publishers, 1997.

SECTION I

# THE EXPERIENCE OF PRACTICE

Chapter 1

# Minding the Body

> An embodied spirituality requires an aesthetic attitude to the world . . . It requires pleasure, joy in the bodily connection with earth and air, sea and sky, plants and animals . . . It is the body that makes spiritual experience passionate, that brings to it intense desire and pleasure, pain, delight, and remorse . . . ; sex and art and music and dance and the taste of food . . . The mechanism by which spirituality becomes passionate is metaphor. An ineffable God requires metaphor not only to be imagined but to be approached, exhorted, confronted, struggled with, and loved.
>
> (Johnson and Lakoff 1999, 566f)

## THE BODY AND THE MIND

It has been claimed elsewhere that the body and movement are not intrinsically important.[1] The body and movement *are* important whether they are attributed meaning at any given moment or not. This assertion may be understood from the anthropological perspective and methodology. In the cultural context, rituals summon liminal states where interpretive meaning is obvious and highly charged to elucidate this very same meaning in everyday contexts. This is why rituals are commonly arenas for learning (through exposure to novel ideas) and the shifting of perceptions on reality. As with a piece of art, they place the focus on meaning by shifting the context to a symbolic frame. This is not, however, meant to suggest that quotidian life is dull and meaningless, but rather that it is rich with meaning, but rarely recognised, since the actions and objects of daily life are understood as functional or practical (rather than interpretive).

Everything can be given greater meaning after being subject to analysis, but one may have powerful experiences that avoid this attribution.

DOI: 10.4324/9781003471752-3

Consider, for example, when one finds pleasure in a work of art, but cannot explain why. The pleasure is real, yet absent analysis, this pleasure may be the by-product of the newness or novelty of the experience alone. This kind of "novelty" (the verbal noun) indicating freshness or the unfamiliar is very different from "novelty" (the noun), that designates something as insignificant, like a trinket. The distinction may not be in the object itself, but in the quality of the experience had by the viewer. In essence, the anthropological method often focuses on the unfamiliar (rituals, festivals, the unusual) in order to reveal significant meaning in the ordinary. To suggest that, without attributed meaning, movement is meaningless is simply to take the often-riddled position that if a tree falls in the forest and no one hears it, it did not make a sound. But the tree *did* make a sound, and movement impacts both the mover as well as those (if any) who witness it.

Historically, yoga philosophy has held different positions on the meaning and function of the living body. During the period in which *haṭha* yoga came to prominence, the body became the central focus of practice. For the medieval Tantric practitioner, the body was seen as the vehicle for enlightenment, for they believed that, unlike deities who exist on an astral plane, human beings, having possession of a body, can seek enlightenment. So important is this embodiment that the *Kulā-Aṃava-Tantra* (1:16-27) chastises those who would fail to take advantage of this opportunity. It notes:

> After obtaining a human body, which is difficult to obtain and which serves as a ladder to liberation, who is more sinful than he who does not cross over to the Self?
>
> Therefore, upon obtaining the best possible life form, he who does not know his own good is merely killing himself.
>
> How can one come to know the purpose of human life without a human body?
>
> One's self is the vessel for everything.
>
> Village, house, land, money, even auspicious and inauspicious karma can be obtained over and over again, but not a human body.
>
> For the purpose of obtaining knowledge, the virtuous purpose should preserve the body with effort. Knowledge aims at the yoga of meditation. He will be liberated quickly.
>
> What fool starts digging a well when his house is already on fire? So long as this body exists, one should cultivate truth.

> One should cultivate the highest good while the senses are not yet frail, suffering is not yet firmly rooted, and adversities have not yet become overwhelming.
>
> (Feuerstein 1998, 53–54)

In order to understand the inner workings of the body that might facilitate the process of self-realisation, the Tantrics devised a metaphorical understanding of the body, consisting of five layers (*koshas*) – ranging from the gross (flesh and bones) to the subtle (state of bliss) with incremental layers of subtlety between (energetic, mind, and discernment). In addition, the *prānamayakośa* (energy body) was imagined as a network of 72,000 energy channels (*nāḍīs*) which extended outside of the body, of which three were important to the process of energy movement. At the crossroads of this tangle of *nāḍīs* were hubs of a sort called *cakras* (of various numbers, in different texts) and knots (*granthis*). The process of liberation or self-realisation entailed the movement of energy (*kuṇḍalinī*) in specific ways from the base of the spine, through these congested hubs and knots to the crown of the head, thereby joining opposing forces, imagined as feminine (*śakti*) and masculine (*śiva*) energy. This understanding of the structure of the body most likely arose out of experiments devised from experiences the *haṭha* yogis were already having rather than from philosophies of the body themselves, since the body has no choice but to move and react to the experience of these movements. This was known as well to the meditative yogis who sought to still the natural and inevitable movement of the living and everchanging body in order to mimic the stillness and unchangingness of the divine energy with which they sought to merge. The theory of merging was based on the foundational observation that a definitive characteristic of the body is that it moves. In other words, the theories of bodily structure evolved from the process of making sense of bodily experiences and not from attempts to abstractly conceptualise the meaning of the body.

Religious scholar Loriliai Biernaki states in her analysis of *bhāvana* and *vikalpa* that imagination has connections with the body, specifically within the context of contemplative practices. She looks to the texts from the 10th and 11th century philosophical school of the Pratyabhijñā of Abhinavagupta and Utpaladeva to show that there are two kinds of imagination, one embodied (*bhāvana*), and one not (*vikalpa*). This association distinguishes between imaginative processes that are useful to contemplative endeavours (specifically yoga) and those that are not:

> Bhāvana references the imagination in a way that relies upon being embodied, using the sensory capacities available to bodies. Rather than transcending the body, bhāvana uses the body in meditation practices and extends the body through its stereotyped physicality into a conception of

> body as a subtle body (puryaṣṭaka, sūkṣma śarīrā, liṅga śarīra) . . . On the other hand, the term vikalpa points to the kind of imagination that generates objects through breaking things down into their parts and rearranging. This type of imagination relies on a multiplication of binaries that sees the world in opposing categories. Vikalpa works against the soteriological aims of meditative practice . . . .
>
> (Biernacki 2017, 2)

Gerrit Lange looking at the history of orthodox Hindu contemplative practices (including yoga) concludes that interactions with the sacred are more often than not embodied. Ritual seeks a mystical encounter that is direct and physical. These experiences are often described in terms of intense feelings of heat and emotional states which range from fear to ecstasy. As he states:

> . . .[Worship] is often aiming at emotional encounter or even identification with specific deities . . . [It] forms the background to study religious storytelling as a part of religious practices – one way to embody and feel religion. A complementary task, then, is to look within the stories for what they tell about bodies and feelings.
>
> (Lange 2022, 2)

What these studies and many like them reveal are that contemplative and mystical experience, whether imaginative or made "real", were viewed as functions of human's corporeal nature.

The one thing that human beings across time, space, and culture have in common is that they all reside in human bodies that move in similar ways. As stated, it is more likely therefore, that the underlying goals and processes of yoga arose from within these bodily experiences rather than the other way around and that these goals and processes have changed according to the changing analyses of these bodily experiences – what were/are relevant and practical endeavours at a particular time and place. The techniques of yoga lend themselves to a variety of goals and these goals are ever changing. Regardless of the speculation that inevitably accompanies the discussion of the origins of yoga and the particulars of its methodology, one can safely say that the body is both a central concern and important to theory and practice.

## EMBODIMENT AND THE BODY

The foundational importance of the body and movement can also be illustrated from the research in many modern disciplines. Contrary to the privileging of mind over body premised by Cartesian duality, researchers suggest that the body and its kinetic interactions are the source material for understanding the nature of reality. As anthropologist Thomas Csordas states, " . . .the body is not an *object* to be studied in relation to culture, but it is to be considered as the *subject* of culture, or in other words, as the existential ground of culture" (Csordas 1990, 5–47). Additionally, psychologist Mark Johnson in *The Body in the Mind* explores the ways that meaning, understanding, and rationality arise from, and are conditioned by, the patterns of our bodily experience (Johnson 1987, 159). As Johnson states of the significance of his work:

> I have tried to show how patterns of sensorimotor interactions are a basis for the meaning of concrete concepts and then how imaginative processes like conceptual metaphor make it possible for us to do all of our most amazing feats of abstract reasoning, from moral deliberation to politics to logic.
> (Johnson 2008)

According to Csordas and Johnson, the body is never inconsequential. It is either the reason we seek meaning (Csordas' existential ground of culture) or the basis for it (Johnson's bodily experience creating knowledge). Whichever the body's role, it is clear that it must be considered in any understanding of human experience, and that through movement, bodies interact with and explore their environment to make sense of reality. Likewise, in the *Phenomenology of Perception*, philosopher Maurice Merleau-Ponty states that the body "can symbolize existence because it brings it into being and actualizes it" (Merleau-Ponty 1978, 158–408). He goes on to say that " . . . the thickness of the body, far from rivaling that of the world, is on the contrary the sole means I have to go into the heart of the things, by making myself a world and by making them flesh" (Merleau-Ponty 1968, 138). It is only through experiences in the body that one interacts with and creates a version of the world and a version of oneself within it. We are, according to Merleau-Ponty, the product of our unique lived experience in our unique bodies.

In *The Primacy of Movement*, philosopher Maxine Sheets-Johnson also proclaims the essential nature of the body and movement. Her wide ranging and eclectic analysis takes an evolutionary perspective on the importance of the body in all acts of consciousness, but in particular in its essential role in both feelings and emotional responses. She draws on the work of scholars in a variety of disciplines (Darwin [1965], Bull [1951], Giggs [2006], Jacobson [1970]) to instantiate her claims that movement is a foundational form of communication and meaning making (the only one available to infants before they master language) and is at the root of consciousness. As she states:

> Without the readiness to act in a certain way, without certain corporeal tonicities, a certain feeling would not, and indeed, could not be felt, and a

> certain action would not, and indeed, could not be taken, since the postural dynamics of the body are what make the feeling and the action possible.
> (Sheets-Johnson 2001, 265)

The basic principle of the theory expressed in experimental findings and clinical practice is that neuromuscular tension is emotionally laden; "neuromuscular acts participate in mental activities . . . including emotions" (Jacobson 1970, 34. From Sheets-Johnson 2001, 26). "Postural attitude" – the tonality needed in the body to ready oneself to express an emotion, a necessary substratum of action, is a prerequisite for movement and therefore emotion. For example, for one to *feel* angry, one inevitably will first assume a postural attitude through which anger can be expressed. There may be a tightening of the chest and a clenching of the jaw. This tonicity creates a feeling which is then interpreted as anger, an interpretation which may be acted upon or inhibited (each requiring their own effort). Therefore, according to Sheets-Johnson, there are no thoughts absent the emotional content predicated by postural attitude, and neither are there the strong motivations to move or act.

Literary critic Susan Sontag also alludes to the visceral nature of meaning in her seminal work, *Against Interpretation.* She writes of the arts, that "to interpret is to impoverish, to deplete the world – in order to set up a shadow world of 'meanings'". She appeals to what she terms an "*ecstasy of surrender*" rather than depending on interpretation as meaning and avers that "[i]n place of a hermeneutics we need an *erotics* of art" (Sontag 1966). These allusions to *ecstasy* and *erotics* distinguish *meaning* from *interpretation* – meaning is rooted in bodily experience and interpretation is the intellectualising of the mind. Arguing within the dualistic understanding of mind and body, Sontag suggests that meaning made through purely cerebral pursuits pales in comparison to experience. Meaning is a fundamental reaction to bodily experience – as with our reaction to viewing a novel piece of art. Interpretation is the process of creating a narrative of these sensorial experiences. It tells a story which later might be seen as an explanation or theory.[2]

## POSTURAL ATTITUDE AND YOGA POSTURES

"Postural attitude" should not be confused with yoga "postures". Postures are shapes that have no intrinsic meaning, though they may be performed with an "attitude" that attributes meaning by using the imagination. Postures are meant however, to have an inherent "balance" in performance. This may be why *āsana* (translated as "stable seat") is usually described in traditional doctrine as a seated posture. A stable seat was either least likely to be subject to external forces which might create a bodily reaction that begs response, or possibly, the adept was tasked with working to maintain a balance that prevented external forces from unsettling them. In any case, a posture may "create" an attitude, that may result in a bodily response of tonicity, but this will depend on how the practitioner executes the posture. If one performs a warrior pose "confidently" with the chest raised and expanded, for example, this may cause a subtle bodily response that "feels" powerful. The body is a tool for discovery – postural attitude is the body's reaction to stimuli, that generates emotional content, that encourages the desire to move in a certain way and is necessarily a precursor to creating and expressing meaning. For *vinyāsa* yoga practitioners, who are constantly in smooth, flowing motion, this idea may have already been discovered in practice. It is through the ever-changing nature of the experience of movement that one is able to reveal the world breath by breath. While moving, one simultaneously uses imagination to create metaphorical understandings of their complex experiences.

The spotlight of our consciousness, which here engages in analysis and forms conclusions, is a very narrow frame. It privileges the mind as the arbiter of reality, consigning the body to a mere dwelling place for this independent mind. While those opposing this duality may argue that attempts to distinguish the body and mind misrepresent the dynamics of meaning making, embodiment theory across disciplines has forcefully questioned the efficacy of these dualistic theoretical positions and sought to prove that the body and bodily experience actually create the mind (Merleau-Ponty 1978). The body motivates analysis, and in this analysis, the narrower frameworks of interpretation are generated. It is *meaning* that originates in the lived experience of the body and leads to the analytic and interpretive speculation that we evolve into explanations and theories. With the knowledge that this is an unsettled question, how should a practitioner use yoga techniques to evolve? One way is to see everything as potentially interesting; to explore without investment in confirming one's beliefs.

## NARCISSISM, VANITY, AND YOGIC SKILL

A common critique in the contemporary yoga academic literature is that "the scene" has become debased by an overemphasis on the physical – an emphasis that is seen to diminish the loftier, spiritual dimensions of practice. There may, indeed, be much that is accurate in such a description. There may, however, be unfair presumptions underlying this conclusion. One such presumption is that the body is not instrumental in spiritual pursuit; it is a cage enmeshing and entangling the soul with the tether of materiality and only by its elimination can the soul be set free. Is the body – and the senses which are the instruments used to interpret its relationship with the world – so wholly antithetical to spiritual development? Does indulgence in the delights of the physical pollute the purity of consciousness? If "all is one", why would the body – the physical – not be an apt receptacle for that oneness to be expressed?

When the body is seen as an obstacle, those who focus on bodily development are seen as shallow or vain rather than self-confident or disciplined. The vain are believed to be focused on physical improvement to the detriment of any higher ends, but on the contrary, many are motivated to self-improvement, and this may be an inspiration to achieve loftier goals. Self-confidence is not the same as the high degree of self-centeredness found in narcissism; for narcissism has much broader implications. Narcissism is a pathology and vanity is a form of self-approbation. In the yoga world, the subject of body positivity emanating from this perspective has led to the ethos of, "whatever you look like is perfect". But is bodily acceptance any less vain a mindset than bodily improvement? In both instances, the body and its appearance are the focus of practice – in contrast to what one might call "body neutrality", where the body's appearance is viewed as inconsequential and left unexamined. In the first case, the practitioner aims at some level to improve their body. This may be purely for aesthetic reasons, but it could also be practical – the body must be fit enough to explore the nature of reality in somatic practice (Sinh 1997, 76). In the second case, the practitioner is still focused on their body – but this is simply an act of self-love or self-acceptance. There is no other practicality to it. Without reproach, practitioners are encouraged to work on their minds for spiritual development but not their bodies. As Loriliai Biernaki concludes in her discussion of tantric conceptions of *bhāvana* (embodied imagination) mentioned above:

> The purveyors of yoga in the West have leaned on a model of yoga as transcendence instead of this "easy path" of embodiment that Utpaladeva gives, perhaps precisely because of a still embedded incommensurable split between mind and body in the contemporary West.
>
> (Biernacki 2017, 12)

## NOVELTY, INSPIRATION, AND WISDOM

The myth of the heroic artist/creator may draw upon the notion that they invent from nothing something that is vibrantly affective and original. As such, they are given preferential status – their patrons, be they kings or wealthy businesspeople – may deferentially hold their ladders or brushes and palette. Yet, this myth misses out on the manner in which inspiration is more often found by discovering something that is partly hidden, or merely suggested from degraded information – as we might see the shape of an animal in clouds or a landscape in a water stain on a white wall. The artist might study stains or swirling mists to discover, through their random forms, something latent. In this sense, it is discovered rather than invented. The scene that this Rorschach style of creation evokes: is it with the wall stain or is the thing discovered within the artist? Conceivably, it is in the relationship of the two. Without the stimulus, the artist would not come up with that particular vision, so, it is somewhat within the stain. At the same time, no two artists would come up with the identical vision; it is uniquely something from within the artist. The inspiration is not something that can be predicted through codified procedures; rather, it can only be courted by providing circumstances in which it may happen.

A quick trawl through Instagram, Facebook, and TikTok yoga posts will likely find numerous mentions of inspiration, said in reference to splendidly executed postures, pictures of nature, or even in philosophic insight. What is the role of inspiration in modern yoga practice and where might it go in the future? At its most simple, people who enjoy moving and who enjoy seeing what bodies are capable of doing, will take delight in seeing others execute material well and may feel "inspired" to work harder on their own practice. This they may do in imitation of another's form, or it may lead to experimentation with the details they admire. There are those in modern yoga who are particularly eager to "invent" new postures, and new fusions of yoga with other movement styles and even improbable fusions – yoga and CBD, goat yoga, and yoga and wine. They "invent" new places where yoga can be practiced, well outside of traditional contexts – corporate cafeterias, church basements, prisons, farms, and animal shelters. But how much is invented – conjured from nothing – and how much is a development from a recognisable starting point? In any case, practitioners are quite enamoured with these novel creations and will likely seek out teachers who they believe are novel as well.

What is lost when novelty is sought rather than experience or expertise? One grows *wise* through experiences over time. Traditionally, the practice of yoga was thought to produce 'wisdom' – deep, transcendent self-knowledge and an understanding of universal truth and cosmic ontology (Alter 2020, 103). Wisdom is not the same as knowledge or intelligence. Intelligence is one's capability to learn and understand, and knowledge is information acquired through learning. Wisdom entails taking into account the wholeness and contradictory nature of things. Wisdom involves deep insight based on experience that is more profound than knowledge or understanding that is simply learned, shared, and communicated. As Joseph Alter states:

> Wisdom is . . . the idealization of an idea about the relationship among general knowledge, truth, and self-awareness. It is a cultural phenomenon.

> As such, what counts as wisdom is variable depending on context, even though in many contexts the terms and conditions of wisdom are thought to be universal . . . Wisdom most certainly has a social foundation in the sense that a person must be recognized as wise by someone else. No matter how reflexive or introspective, wisdom does not exist in isolation from a community, and, in some sense, consensus is the foundation upon which wisdom is culturally constructed.
>
> (Alter 2020, 106)

In yoga today, wisdom may refer to a means of personal transformation; of expanding our consciousness in the ways we understand and relate to our world. But wisdom traditions are not just resident in a person – they are traditions of thought which exist at the level of community.[3] Quite a fuss may be made of the importance of the "wisdom of the ancestors", the great yogis who seemed to know all the answers – knowledge that may have been lost, but if rediscovered will show us the path to enlightenment. Whatever way it is defined, the meaning and importance of wisdom in any community will be reflected in the ways in which it shapes and takes shape in practice. This wisdom is different from knowledge in that it is trusted and therefore, not readily questioned. Looking at contemporary yoga practice, one sees a growing rejection of the kind of status differences that wisdom endowed upon the *gurus* of the past, and a distrust of the wholehearted dedication and faith the *śiṣya* (disciple) placed in such *gurus* (teachers). Theodora Wildcroft suggests that, more likely, the trend is toward "post-lineage yoga", where practitioners are their own *gurus* seeking their own wisdom through their own experiences with people like themselves (Wildcroft 2018). Whatever the role for wisdom of the *guru* in contemporary yoga, practitioners are seeking novel experiences of their own without its endorsement. But this may not mean that wisdom is no longer valued, simply that in the future, the community that endorses and values it may shift away from historical toward contemporary worldviews.

## NOVELTY AND THE FRAME

If the frame placed around a picture sets the perimeter within which one might entertain an interpretation or find a new perspective, this is, in part, due to the fact that the literal frame assumes a "symbolic frame". This symbolic frame both defines the parameters of interpretation and indicates that the interpretation will not be literal. Once a painting of a tree is placed in a frame, it requires a symbolic interpretation, it is neither paint on canvas nor simply a tree. Instead, an interpretation is encouraged, if not demanded, that will reveal something unique to each individual who views it. Within this symbolic context, one is free to play with novel ideas – to entertain a different set of values, beliefs, and ideals. In essence, one is able to assess their cultural beliefs and alter them through this window to new interpretation – if they are seeking knowledge and understanding. This is how, contrary to Sontag's presumed views, interpretation can bolster one's appreciation of novel experience – it offers opportunities for innovation. When art is particularly challenging, it generally expresses meaning that is contrary to one's perceived reality. In this way, one sees the power of culture to influence interpretation, but also the individual's ability to surpass/transcend their current worldview. It is not that Sontag is misguided in her affection for sheer experience, it is that the "interpretation" she imagines comes purely from outside the individual, rather than being a dynamic between the individual, their culture, and the sensual experience. What Sontag (1966) argues against is the rigid imposition of a frame or theory that dictates interpretation without valuing the unique and necessary input of the individual.

One of the reasons *vinyāsa* yoga[4] should provide a particularly good context for novel meaning making (the altering of worldview) is that it insists on the constancy of change and values the sensory information offered by reality as expressively neutral. Novel experience is of particular interest because when new values and ideas are presented, one engages with something other than themselves and may be altered as one enters new territory of experience and understanding. Sensory interaction is the engagement with the Other (Csordas' "kinetic interactions") and creates internal imagery. The interpretation of this imagery may reveal the Self to the self – evoking rejection (a doubling down of beliefs) or an embrace of the new with a change of ideas. Both rejection and acceptance are a product of reflection upon the actual experience whether it be art or yoga. The rejection assumes that the internal realm of meaning is already correct or well substantiated – that any novel information is less appealing than one's existing internal reality – truer than whatever alternate reality the senses deliver to this inner realm.

The skills required of one who views or appreciates the novel are not the same as those of the creator. In the performing arts, the skill level is generally not meant to intrude on the audience's engagement with the subject matter. This is an important distinction – there are forms of public performances (e.g., acrobatic circus acts) where the audience is meant to be impressed by the spectacular feats of the performers themselves because it is the unusual skill that is novel. There are other kinds of performance (e.g., when an actor or dancer plays the role of a character) where the skill level is meant to remain hidden. For this to work as art, the actor must be subsumed within the character – they must be looked through so that the character remains the object of focus. If the actor achieves a certain level of mastery, their skill level is not a distraction. With this in mind, the yoga practitioner walks an interesting tightrope – they, like the audience, interpret through the senses but are at the same time the artist/creator. For the focus to remain on the experience, the skill level must be so high that it does not draw attention to itself when executing *āsana* or *vinyāsa* – the skill level must be intuitive and unreflective (state of flow). Practitioners of modern yoga are left with a conundrum – how to challenge themselves to master new skills and also have opportunities to experience the state of flow where higher pursuits might be achieved. None of this devalues the body or renders it irrelevant; on the contrary, it exults in the body and the skill level that transforms it into the artist's creation – a rendering of an everchanging and malleable self – a self that is the amalgam of mind and body. They are one with each other (the spiritual and material) in the same way that energy and mass can be equivalent.

## ART, YOGA, AND THE BODY

The fact that yoga postures have no utility makes it possible to creatively attribute different meanings or interpretations to them. But the assumption must always be that whatever construct of that meaning is made, it is meant to have the same kind of provisionality as art – we accept it temporarily to see what such a perspective might reveal, but we do not mistake it for the only *actual* reality. The idea that the person doing the posture is simply "being" – existing in "the present" – is only a superficial appraisal. It is not just so "simple". The practitioner is convincingly playing a person doing postures in a yoga practice. But they are also the sum of their life outside their practice – the niggling injuries, problems at work, and their state of hunger. The yoga class represents a rarified opportunity for studying the body's capacity for meaning making. When provisionally attributing meaning to the movement and positioning of their bodies, the practitioners' focus is on the execution of postures. Postures function as malleable symbols with a variety of expressions.

The problem with philosophies that speculate on consciousness is that as soon as one begins to analyse one begins to objectify and the thing (even one's own consciousness) begins to seem alien. Whereas the lived body has no time to reflect. It is, perhaps, only in the spurt of creativity, when one is in the process of making the posture, that the person exists without the inflections of objective analysis. One becomes the process – energy begetting energy. Before the creating occurs however, there must be conscious intention to set the parameters that frame the creation (its intended meaning). One steps onto their mat and creates a version of themselves as a practitioner and temporarily abandons the trappings of their everyday life. This frees them to experience this slice of reality with their body through yoga. Ideally, the delight of anticipation or the poignancy of regret are relinquished; there is no looking into the past or projecting into the future. There is only the intense and immediate energy of doing. This is a different way of perceiving energy than "Blue is the preferential reflection of a wavelength of light that is 450 – 495 nanometers" which, while precisely accurate in an analytical sense, utterly fails to distinguish what it is like to experience "blue".[5] This seemingly objective quantification of colour neutralises its evocative nature and turns it into something that can be manipulated. This is a shared conceit – that its (blue's) "impression" on the world is contaminative to understanding it's essentiality. Where, in actuality, it is the messiness – the multiplicity – of all that is and all the unpredictable affects which blue produces that *reveal* the chaotic nature of reality. It is through the simplification of art that we can focus in the present on its elusive nature – and recognise that the elusive nature of reality and the transcendent can be revealed through the techniques of physical yoga and art.

## IMPLICATIONS: THE FUTURE IS NOW

### Spirituality and the Necessity of the Body

Physical yoga is understood today as a healthful practice. The designation of yoga as exercise or a vehicle for stress reduction provides it a logical utility. Though health is an important pursuit that serves to justify the physical practice, there are a number of other fitness regimens that can accomplish these same goals, arguably more efficiently. But yoga is also perceived, even by those who practice for healthful reasons, as offering more than physical benefits – yoga has higher, spiritual aims that are attributed to practices perceived to be of the *mind* (e.g., meditation). As Johnson and Lakoff (1999) suggest, however, the body must be the vehicle for spirituality. What is spirituality if not a profound "feeling"? Until teachers and practitioners see their bodies as spiritually essential, physical practice will be relegated to these lesser uses and be accorded lesser value. Most contemporary yoga styles approach practice from a physical perspective and rationalise the conflict between techniques (the physical ones) and the aims of practice (a recognition of a Self that has no karmic entanglement with the world) in two ways. The first is to say that the physical work is merely preparation for the more "advanced" work of *rājā* yoga and the second is to ignore the spiritual dimensions of yoga and claim that it is a health regimen.

"An embodied spirituality requires an aesthetic attitude" (Johnson and Lakoff 1999) and is founded in sensual engagement with the world. It is the essence of spiritual experience, for absent the body, nothing remains but the abstract conceptions of a supposedly untethered mind. It is through the body/mind that one encounters the spirit; it is not a *conception,* but an *experience.* In this era of unprecedented popularity for yoga, it seems extraordinary that embodied spirituality, as a yogic term, should require clarification and examination. It is necessary because, in this era, a large part of the foundation of yoga technique is derived from interpretations of Patañjali's *Yoga Sūtras* (and a reverence for its historicity) and focusses on negating the body; it sees the body as an impediment to achieving spiritual insight and liberation. In short, the body is associated with materiality (almost inescapably tying the yoga aspirant to the world) and the processes of consciousness are deemed spiritual (part of a higher realm). But the feeling of spiritual embodiment (and, in particular, ecstasy) is under-examined in yoga, in large part because such intense and deeply personal experiences are difficult to describe. This is why metaphor is central to an understanding of the ineffable. It is through the body-mind that one encounters the spirit. To articulate spiritual experience as pure conception, therefore, requires metaphor.

The idea that there is an unbroachable divide between materiality and spirituality (or between mind and body) while still maintaining their factual reality sounds like a difficult premise to defend. Its origins may lie in the Samkhyist notion of two categories of utterly independent reality: *prakṛti* and *puruṣa* – the first of which is perishable or transitory and the other which is permanent and unchanging. The material realm of *prakṛti* (which includes the body) is said to have no means of apprehending pure consciousness; the spiritual realm of *puruṣa.* The yoga techniques for attaining this state of pure consciousness, therefore, deal with overcoming or negating the body's influence on perception. But however one construes the idea of spiritual ecstasy, it is something that is *felt* – spiritual ecstasy is embodied and is not meant to be abstract or merely conceptual. It is meant to be experienced or lived before it is understood by giving it meaning.

As yoga evolves, how might we encourage the exploration of spiritual embodiment? One way would be to focus on aesthetic appreciation (the experience of beauty) as embodied and discovered through sensual engagement with the world. By aesthetic appreciation we mean, a refined awareness experienced through deep involvement of the senses – a sensual inhabiting and cultivation of the world. For example, in practicing yoga, a person doing postures experiences beauty by becoming a 3-dimensional moving sculpture – they are, at once, audience, creator, and creation. This would provide an opportunity to practice exploring the physical reality of the experience of "the spirit". Another approach would involve changing the nature of yoga class so as to facilitate the experience of intense spiritual embodiment. This would allow the practitioner to use their skills of aesthetic appreciation to physically express states of spirituality. In most instances, however, public expression of extreme feeling is not encouraged – it is actually frowned upon in yoga contexts unless it is "positive", or upbeat and cheerful, and, importantly, something that does not interfere with the practice of others in class. If Johnson and Lakoff are correct, and spirituality is a highly sensual experience, physical expressions of this experience (like emotional release) must be accepted and even encouraged within the yoga community before it can be fully explored.

At present, relatively inert postures such as corpse pose are associated with the apex of spiritual experience – "the mind floats free of the body" would be a typical metaphor. But if spiritual experience is understood as bodily experience, the future might look to a different framework where the intensity of the *commitment* to the physical experience itself is the indicator of spiritual engagement. This kind of intensity is found in the depth of appreciation of sensual experience (what Sontag [1966] termed the "ecstasy of surrender") and should not be confused with the level of difficulty of postures or sequences or other yogic activities. The activities themselves are not important; it is the way in which the body/mind commits to achieving their liberation. Consider the range of experiences available in a typical yoga class. It is no wonder that practitioners frequently ask their teacher "what am I supposed to feel?". The range and intensity of experiences are limited by the parameters the teacher sets. The emphasis is likely on learning the alignment of postures, sequences, and other skills. There is less opportunity for actually "doing" yoga – being free to have a wide and unpredictable range of sensual/spiritual experience. There is an opportunity to have a profound experience (physical and mental) in all of the practice, but most are saving this "surrender" for *śavāsana.*

Metaphors describing sensual intensity are often touched with sexual inference, and it may be that part of the nature of sexual experience is its apparent potency for liberating the mind through the body – it requires some kind of letting go to the activity to fully experience it. The most overtly yogic achievement – its spiritual consummation – would be a realisation of the unity of reality that can be revealed through *any* sensual information. Eating a peach or hearing a song or seeing a snowy mountain have the same potential to reveal perspective on the Totality. The goal of a physical practice is to realise how spiritual grace and physical grace equate. This is not something that would represent a wholly new awareness. Undoubtedly, great practitioners past and present have also understood that grace is found by employing exactly the right amount of energy to their endeavours. Those who try too hard miss the mark as much as those whose efforts are inadequate. Grace – past, present, and future – can be found in the energetically appropriate.

Still today, the mind/body distinction, best articulated in the West as Cartesian dualism, has reinforced the idea that the body stands in the way of higher endeavours like spiritual development and must be overcome. When yoga philosophy was first introduced to the West by a variety of Indian scholars (most prominently Svāmi Vivekānanda), they sought to aver the sophistication of Eastern philosophy and its tenets. To do so, they adapted yogic principles to Western dualism and framed the body and body practices as corruptions of the purity of thought practiced by Indian scholars and adepts. This presentation of yoga philosophy as a meditative practice was a way to gain power by meeting orientalist expectations – the West with its superior material culture, and the East as spiritually advanced. Today, though many may give lip service to the primacy of the mind/body connection (including ourselves, disappointingly), many still perceive the mind as transcendent and the body as hopelessly tethered to materialism, and act accordingly. How many times have we heard that we are not what is seen on the outside, but what is inside (our mind), even though embodiment theory notes decisively that the sum total of our very different experiences, in our very different bodies, is what *makes* who we are on the inside. If yoga is to evolve to better fulfil spiritual pursuits, its practitioners will have to better question this dualist assumption, and also practice in a way that reveals the importance of the body in the process of enlightenment.

## NOTES

1. In Western culture, the philosophical tenets of Cartesian duality privilege the mind over the body, sometimes to the extent that the body is considered not simply inferior (e.g., a temporary prison for the mind and spirit) but inconsequential.
2. To Christopher Hill "Interpretation is subjective understanding, whereas meaning is the substance of understanding . . . Books provide the understanding of its author, but your understanding of what you read is subjective to your understanding of all other things. So, when you interpret something, it is understood through your perceptive lens" (Foxley 2015, 206).
3. In philosophy, "wisdom traditions" are understood as precepts which are shared by all religions, but uniquely interpreted in each orthodoxy.
4. *Vinyāsa* yoga is a style of physical practice which entails continuous movement impelled by *ujjayi* breath.
5. Example courtesy Iain McGilchrist.

## REFERENCES

Alter, Joseph. 2020. "Yoga and Wisdom: Reflections on the Body at the Intersection of Epistemology and Ontology". In *Capturing the Ineffable: An Anthropology of Wisdom*, edited by Philip Y. Kao and Joseph S. Alter, 103–121. Toronto: University of Toronto Press.

Biernacki, Loriliai. 2017. "Imagining the Body in Tantric Contemplative Practice". *International Journal of Dharma Studies* 5 (4). DOI 10.1186/s40613-016-0043-7.

Bull, Nina. 1951. *The Attitude Theory of Emotion.* First Edition. New York: Nervous and Mental Disease Monographs.

Csordas, Thomas J. 1990. "Embodiment as a Paradigm for Anthropology". *Ethos* 18 (1): 5–47. Accessed 12 March 2023. https://www.jstor.org/stable/640395.

Darwin, Charles (1872/1965). *The Expression of the Emotions in Man and Animals.* Chicago, IL: University of Chicago.

Feuerstein, Georg. 1998. *Tantra: The Path to Ecstasy.* Boston: Shambala.

Foxley, Rachel. 2015. "The Logic of Ideas in Christopher Hill's English Revolution". *Prose Studies: History, Theory, Criticism* 36 (3): 199–208. https://doi.org/10.1080/01440357.2014.994727.

Griggs, S. 2006. "Rational Choice in Public Policy: The Theory in Critical Perspective". In *Handbook of Public Policy Analysis: Theory, Politics and Methods,* edited by Frank Fischer, Gerald J. Miller, and Mara S. Sidney. New York: CRC Press.

Jacobson, Edmund. 1970. *Modern Treatment of Tense Patients.* Springfield, IL: Charles C. Thomas.

Johnson, Mark. 1987. *The Body in the Mind: The Bodily Basis of Meaning, Imagination, and Reason.* Chicago, IL: University of Chicago Press, 1987.

Johnson, Mark. 2008. "What Makes a Body?" *Journal of Speculative Philosophy* 22 (3): 159–169.

Johnson, Mark and George Lakoff. 1999. *Philosophy in the Flesh: The Embodied Mind and Its Challenge to Western Thought.* New York: Basic Books.

Lange, Gerrit. 2022. "Hindu Deities in the Flesh: 'Hot' Emotions, Sensual Interactions, and (Syn)aesthetic Blends". *Religions* 13 (11): 1045. https://doi.org/10.3390/ rel13111045.

Merleau-Ponty, Maurice. 1968. *The Visible and the Invisible.* Translated by Alphonso Lingis. Evanston: Northwestern University Press.

Merleau-Ponty, Maurice. 1978. *Phenomenology of Perception.* London: Routledge & Kegan Paul.

Sheets-Johnson, Maxine. "Emotion and Movement: A Beginning Empirical-Phenomenological Analysis of Their Relationship". *Journal of Consciousness Studies* (2001) 259–277. Accessed 03/12/22. https://www.academia.edu/8548014/Emotion_and_Movement.

Sinh, Pancham, trans. 1997. *The Hāṭha Yoga Pradipīkā,* Fifth Edition. New Dehli: Munshiram Manoharlal Publishers Pvt. Ltd.

Susan Sontag. 1966. *Against Interpretation, and Other Essays.* New York: Farrar, Straus & Giroux.

Wildcroft, Theadora. 2018. "Patterns of Authority and Practice Relationships in Post Lineage Yoga" *PhD Thesis,* London: The Open University.

Chapter 2

# Anger is an Energy

> Here all the identification-images are seen as possessed by a violent passion, both wrathful and sexual, symbolizing the extremest [sic] state of aroused energy. After this series of states has been passed through, the mind becomes open to the entire range of possible vision . . . .
>
> (Rawson 1973, 29)

When we "feel", we record sensation. Emotions colour and give contour to the meaning of these feelings especially when the direction of stimuli is from the external world. Antonio Damasio suggests emotions convey the registering of these and colour it so that the direction tends to be outward as a motor responses. Redness in the face, a feeling in the stomach, and rapid heart rate are emotional responses to the feeling or sensation (Damasio 2000, 35–81). This may seem an inadequate accounting for the complexity of feelings, but suffice to say, emotions do exert control over the body; they are corporealised – experienced and processed physically (Csikszentmihalyi 1990).[1] These emotional responses are a way that human beings experience the meaning of their bodies in relation to other objects and persons in the world (phenomenology). Culture also conditions the expression of emotion and its meaning. For example, the British are often described as having a "stiff upper lip", especially when compared to Italians who are seen as "highly expressive". It is not that the British feel less (or that Italians feel more), but simply that each culture prescribes a different way to react to and express these feelings.

## INTENSITY OF EMOTION

In normal contexts, at a certain level of intensity, felt emotional responses may be difficult to differentiate. Joy and grief may both be expressed

DOI: 10.4324/9781003471752-4

through tears. Attraction and aversion might be difficult to distinguish when passions run high. Yet, some yoga teachers attempt to prescribe emotional responses for their students in the context of studio culture. For example, "back bends are joyful because they open the heart and eliminate energetic blockages", and "hip openings liberate pent up trauma and, if properly performed, may result in significant emotional release". According to some styles, injury may result from resistance to these prescribed emotional responses (Sugarman 2022). Students are generally meant to experience strong "positive" emotions and/or sensations in an effort to evoke a "spiritual" response. This may be accomplished through the performance of extreme postures because they are sensorially unambiguous – the teacher assigns emotional meaning to these sensations, and this meaning is contextualised as spirituality. This intensity is experienced as powerful and is interpreted through the culture of the studio as spiritual authenticity (intensity = power = authenticity); an interpretation which removes emotional ambiguity. Through the control of meaning, students' emotional life is given clarity. The sharing of intense experience results in a sense of connection and an alteration of the sense of self based in part on this connection.[2] The intensity of sensation also signifies an investment for students – if one has felt something passionately, it is cherished, and this allows one to overlook faults and pitfalls of their chosen practice. The high investment, coupled with managed emotional clarity and passionately felt sensations, explains why people may remain faithful to *gurus* who have fallen or yoga styles that are unhealthy or unproductive for them.

Strong emotion can also act as a dis-inhibitor because of the diminishing control and volatility one experiences with emotional intensity. Intense emotions require interpretation, although this interpretation may be dynamic. As Saint Teresa of Avila notes in her experience of the ecstasy of divine union:

> In his hands I saw a great golden spear, and at the iron tip there appeared to be a point of fire. This he plunged into my heart several times so that it penetrated to my entrails. When he pulled it out, I felt that he took them with it, and left me utterly consumed by the great love of God. The pain was so severe that it made me utter several moans. The sweetness caused by this intense pain is so extreme that one cannot possibly wish it to cease, nor is one's soul then content with anything but God. This is not a physical, but a spiritual pain, though the body has some share in it – even a considerable share.
>
> (Lewis 2009, Chapter XXIX, Part 17)

The disinhibition and instability resulting from the experience of intense emotion may result in the morphing of emotional meaning and the transfer of these emotions from one person to another. The more intense the emotional response, the more contagious it may become. In a class setting (as with any ritual), emotions are often transferred from one practitioner to another, a sort of 'groupfeel' (analogous to 'groupthink'). This could be the spontaneous shared euphoria of one person's accomplishment, the deliberate insinuation of prescribed emotion (e.g., bliss) by a member of the group or the teacher, or even the collective annoyance felt when someone violates the etiquette of the practice space. The exact meaning of the emotional response need not be clarified since the intensity alone, when physically experienced, is enough to instigate transference. Though emotions are shared, they do not need to mean the same thing to each individual. The need for ongoing interpretation creates a curiosity for those bound up in the 'groupfeel', as with the mystic St. Teresa who seeks to describe the ineffable nature of rapture by sharing the feeling of it. As she goes on to state, "So gentle is this wooing which takes place between God and the soul that if anyone thinks I am lying, I pray God in his goodness, to grant him some experience of it" (Lewis 2009, Chapter XXIX, Part 17).

## HARNESSING CURIOSITY

Curiosity may be understood as the intellectual aspect of emotional or sensorial arousal and is a useful tool in yogic explorations. Yet, curiosity is curtailed in a yoga class where there is a distinction made between "positive" and "negative" emotions. This distinction is a purely cultural one; emotions are *emotions*; they are neither good nor bad and giving them value is a construction based on shared conceptions and beliefs. In Western Culture (and Western yoga practice), positive emotions are generally considered desirable and negative emotions are disparaged. Joy, compassion, or love are valued over anger, frustration, or hate. That negative emotions are viewed pejoratively masks the fact that they are a potent fuel for change – creativity may result from these same emotions. Positive emotions are less likely to demand a response because they represent a desirable state (despite that they are also transitory). The attempt by teachers to prescribe sustained positive emotional response attenuates the students' need for independent reasoning and may hamper their curiosity.

While appropriate emotional response is encouraged on the one hand, the inability to control one's emotions is disparaged in the modern yoga studio. It is seen as a failure of equanimity. In Western culture, emotional expression is equated with a lack of control, weakness, or failure of character. Those who cannot control their emotions are seen as unable to exert control over their world which is considered basic to power. Here, as with intensity, a metaphorical equation is made between emotional control and the ability to exert power. Paradoxically, this presupposes that the only enlightened response is to meet each situation with contentment (evenness of mind). This is also found in the therapeutic practice of radical acceptance (DBT method)[3] where one is trained to meet all events with this self-same evenness – an emotional expression of the acceptance of reality. A practitioner is expected to be "in the moment", yet certain emotional reactions are proscribed. Yoga is also sold as a vehicle for the release of toxins and toxic relationships (that are equated with emotions) rather than through their containment. Because these unwanted emotions are believed to be stored in the physical body, postures and movements are employed as a way to safely discharge them. Positive emotions (respect, contentment, joy, bliss, love, and happiness) are said to result from the accomplishment of this release (Sugarman 2022).

## REACTION AND RESPONSE

To understand the complexity of emotions and their expression, a distinction can be made between 'reaction' and 'response'. When one reacts to an experience reflexively, it is defined in this analysis as reaction. But if one consciously processes sensorial or cognitive information and mitigates their actions accordingly, it is defined as response. Because reactions are spontaneous and immediate, they can be easily associated with the experience of being in the moment. However, in yoga circles, spontaneous joy is valorised, whereas spontaneous anger is not. The sentiment that anger, or so-called negative emotions, are inherently bad denies that they can be responses when they are reasoned rather than reactive. The conscious processing (response) may also be considered "in the moment", as with *vinyāsa*,[4] where one is aware of the movement from moment to moment and is also cognisant of the emotional trajectory as it evolves. Therefore, negative emotions can be as potentially productive for the seeking of equanimity because the energy they produce may be channelled in the service of conscious yogic exploration. The problem is that anger, as an energy, without some kind of conscious processing, may be expressed as an inchoate frustration, which is dispersive of its energetic potential.

In contemporary yoga, primacy has been given to the idea that yoga should make us feel euphoric (to attain a state of bliss). If emotional response is curtailed by prescription to something like "contentment" or "peace of mind" or "self-acceptance", what is the consequence of this muting of emotional response to the intensity of experience? One may find an intense challenge in changing a habit or being still or even being soft; intensity does not necessarily require rigorous physicality or special acrobatic ability. However, the culture-bound feel-good ethos found in contemporary yoga has resulted in emphasis being placed on the finite accomplishments that yoga achieves (e.g., executing a posture, lowering blood pressure, destressing, preserving youthfulness, improving flexibility, helping one sleep, or coping with trauma). Little is said about how emotional responses might fuel more lofty goals. Lofty explorations were likely the concern of the ancients, and their investigations led to a certitude about the infinite nature of reality and its unity, something that could be described emotionally as 'rapture'. Should modern practitioners be prohibited from using the fuel provided by intense emotions to seek the exhilaration found in such investigation, even if this does not result in a "good" feeling?

## RAPTURE

Rapture is a state that attends and responds to the Other in a highly focused way. It is an encounter with the transcendence of possibility. Common examples of enrapt behaviour are found in experiencing nature and viewing works of art. These are states where external forces stimulate innovative internal responses – they are beyond positive and negative. Rapture is a dynamic interaction between the practitioner and the Other that results in a variety of phenomena which affect the body/mind. Tingling, feelings of power, lightness of being, and intimations of the infinite are all examples of the altered sense of self generated through the experience of rapture.

Initial encounters with rapture are usually inadvertent and fortuitous. However, the yogi seeks to find this state deliberately. The yogi creates techniques that are used to attain, sustain, and summon rapture at will. Though it is conceded that rapture might happen unintentionally and without extreme effort (as in coming upon the scenic in nature), it is something that is typically facilitated in yoga through a measure of extremity or intensity (Csikszentmihalyi 1990).[5] This may be because intensity provokes a strong emotional response that is associated with the fixing of memory. The retrieval of memory is facilitated by the repetition of the intense physical experience. This is one of the rationales for studying so-called "advanced" postures. The difficulty of inverted postures and the ability to master them becomes associated with an emotional state of accomplishment in the face of considerable risk. The risk is what seems to make it particularly emotionally resonant. Yoga then inverts this premise and seeks to find within even the simplest movements, a depth of involvement and commitment that would be typically associated with the exceedingly difficult, so that it is the emotion that makes it interesting, not the physical difficulty.

Obtaining a degree of mastery is in itself satisfying, but this satisfaction with one's capability is distinct from rapture. To become enamoured with the accomplishment of physical skills might be an impediment to the development of deeper emotional or imaginative engagement if the skill is seen as an end in and of itself. The pursuit of rapture requires that one overcome complacency; that the ambition of one's striving is not subordinate to, or dependent on, the mastery of physical skills. Intense emotional stimulation helps to invent self-realisation since our sense of self is *created* through emotional experience and the memories created through these emotional responses (Grosz 2014).

## CHANNELLING EMOTION

Today, music is frequently used in the context of practice possibly because music can make the class more emotionally resonant. Music functions in a way that sets the mood or evokes certain feelings because it has an emotional narrative in its 'script'. The practitioner responds to this narrative and generates feelings or emotions within themselves. Similarly, the use of incense, soft lighting, and even heat can be employed to evoke sensorial engagement and enhance the experience of flow while giving significance to the meaning of the experience (Nevrin 2008, 113–139).

According to Csikszentmihalyi:

> 'flow' is a single-minded immersion that represents the ultimate experience of harnessing the emotions in the service of performing and learning. In flow, emotions are not just contained and channelled, but are positive, energised, and aligned with the task at hand. To be caught in the ennui of depression or the agitation of anxiety is to be barred from flow.
>
> (Csikszentmihalyi 1990)

When emotions are reactions rather than responses, their power is unsettling instead of productive. "The hallmark of flow is a feeling of spontaneous joy, even rapture, while performing a task" (Csikszentmihalyi 1990). Flow state is found in yoga practice when the body is controlled by giving it meaningless tasks (*āsana*, *vinyāsa* sequences, *mudrā*, *māntra*) that are formalised as *ritual.*[6] As these shapes and movements have no inherent meaning, the practitioner (or the teacher/ritual operator) creates their own interpretation. There is an ongoing reciprocal relationship between the receiving of physical sensation and the generation of physical sensation through motor response. These are the raw materials through which meaning is created and integrated. Emotions, positive or negative, are not necessarily impediments to advancement; when channelled, they are a powerful and easily accessible fuel for creativity and meaning making.

Emotions allow us to understand the abstract. This is as true for yogic endeavours as it is in everyday life.

## MODERN MYSTICS

The emotional and imaginative content of most contemporary yoga classes is becoming increasingly limited. Studio etiquette requires that emotional responses such as anger and frustration (though still felt) are generally proscribed and nominally replaced by concepts such as self-approval (to self) or loving kindness (to others). There is little opportunity for the grappling with intense emotional meaning of mystical traditions of the past. Unlike St. Teresa, we find little opportunity for the experience of ecstasy, as ironically, spirituality has been made distinct from physical experience. The mystics of the past found spirituality akin to sexual ecstasy – they sought an erotic union with the divine. Perhaps beginning with the heralding of the *Yoga Sūtras of Patañjali* (by Svāmi Vivekānanda) to the West, meditative (cerebral rather than bodily) pursuits have come to be seen as the end goal of spiritual merging. *Haṭha* yoga and other physio-spiritual practices are presented as diversions from the path toward enlightened bliss, delegitimising the intense physical experience once acknowledged by mystics in spiritual union.

Much effort goes into establishing yoga as a serious practical endeavour – a transmissible system of health, fitness, and stress reduction. The vast imaginative and mystical possibilities of cosmic consciousness are now constrained by reliance on quantified proofs of the healthful efficacy of yoga practice. This comes about, in part, through regimentation and conformity – mats in rows, set and unvarying sequences of postures, predetermined ratios for breathing in and out, and the subduing and prescription of emotion are some obvious examples. These do have their uses – very explicit information and experience can be more easily conveyed when the parameters for observation and participation are clearly delineated. Yet, this also narrows the range of acceptable experience and its expression. This should not suggest however, that emotional or imaginative exercises or development be without structure, but that procedures that either prohibit or narrow our range of experience also limit ambition. Emotional and imaginative exploration allow for a broader and more fluid interpretation and discovery of the self. Other physical disciplines – particularly the performing arts – build notions of a malleable (rather than foundational) self into their training. One is invited to be a character – someone other than oneself – whose portrayal is executed by each person in their own unique way. Yoga, on the other hand, has inadvertently confined its acceptable expressions of self to ways that exclude the possibility of ecstatic experiences such as those had by mystics like St. Teresa. Previous generations have construed some intense experiences as mystical in nature and have seen this form of altered consciousness as communion with God. In studio etiquette of the 21st century, this behaviour is implausible. Spiritual possession or ecstasy lie outside of the remit of data driven scientific explanations. The stimuli for rapture are still much the same (e.g., scenic natural settings, works of art, the smell of a baby's skin, the touch of a lover) – situations that induce feelings of awe, wonder, fear, insignificance, inclusion, and connection that are inexplicit yet powerful – and are experienced by the body through the medium of the senses. While the mundane goals of health and wellbeing are laudable, their emphasis has come at the expense of intense emotional and imaginative exploration.[7]

As St. Teresa bemoaned, it is a frustrating challenge to write about the ineffable and what it is to have experiences that transcend the explicit or the quantifiable. James Hewitt observed that if orgasm was an experience that could only be obtained once or twice in a lifetime, it would have spawned great religions to revere (or try to explain) this intense or perhaps gloriously ecstatic feeling – so far beyond the mundane (Hewitt 1991, 502). Indeed, the Tantrics that practised *maithuna* saw sexual arousal as a goad to physically incarnating the nature of the universe – where the participants did so as personifications of gods. In the 21st century, we might wonder why such an overtly human behaviour as sex needs to be explained, or validated, or made authentic by assuming the role of a god. It is just as remarkable and sensorially amazing if one does it as a human. But the verbal description of what intense pleasure feels like remains, at best, a mere shadow of the physical experience – it is within the physical body where the experience of ecstasy lies.

So, is there a way that yoga can be used to feel the pleasure of what used to be called a mystical experience? Or is this potential to be consigned to the waste bin of vain desires and attachments antithetical to loftier pursuits? It seems that the practise of physical yoga techniques (as opposed to motionless meditation technique) are likely to continue. The rationale that *āsana* practice is merely preparation for meditation remains an unproven premise. Rather, *āsana* seems to have more in common with the physical practices associated with mystical experience in many traditions. Aesthetic practices that challenge stamina, endurance of pain, and sustained concentration are found amongst the Sufi dervishes, *Saṃnyāsin* (Tantric) yogis, Hasidic Kabbalists, and charismatic Christians. Should modern yogis look to find spiritual expression through physical experience as well – through a recognition of the physicality of emotional response and its power to explore the sensorial nature of ecstatic experience? The assigning of acceptable emotions by the teacher or a member of the group, only hampers this exploration[8] for it removes the practitioner from the process of meaning making through which consciousness is created. Exploration requires the concerted effort of the practitioner as they, with focused concentration, construct their own "feeling of what happens" (Damasio 2000) – the dynamic unfolding of the internal and external sensations of bodily experience.

## IMPLICATIONS: THE FUTURE IS NOW

According to Asma and Gabriel (2019) emotion is intrinsic to all meaning. They propose that the process of meaning making begins with sensory input creating feelings. At the next level, these feelings are expressed as emotions. Here, experience stored in memory allows for a heightened and individual interpretation of emotional response. At the tertiary level, emotions are interpreted through cultural conventions, refining the meaning. Emotions are malleable and mutable and may be either enhanced or dissuaded though contextualisation (experience) and narration (culture and imagination). This may be why the ancient yogis saw emotions as highly problematic. They were not part of the unchanging foundational reality to which they aspired and, therefore, an impediment to the search for eternal truths about the nature of Self and reality. But research suggests that emotional systems are central to understanding the evolution and function of the human mind through a feedback system that may enlist all three of the strata of meaning making. Therefore, the somatic experience, especially in movement, becomes a central concern in any understanding of consciousness. For the ancients, who sought to imitate what they saw as the immutable and unchanging nature of reality through attempts at stillness, this was meant to result in a concomitant "cessation of the modifications, or fluctuations, of the mind" (*Yoga Sūtras of Patāñjali*, 1.2). For modern yogis, whose practice is more likely characterised by physical engagement and movement in what is believed to be an ever-changing reality, the encounter with consciousness is more complex and dynamic and requires an understanding of cognitive processes. If one agrees that emotions play a role in creating cognition and/or consciousness, then the yoga practitioner of the future should critically examine emotions and their role in these processes.

Other disciplines have found ways to include intense emotion into their training methods and their performance outcomes. The most obvious of these is the theatre where emotional range and authenticity are seen as requisite and learning how these are expressed and repeated is a part of the training and the presentation. No one is upset when profound emotion is experienced because there is an understanding that when the director calls for the action to cease, everyone stops. More than this, it is understood that the emotion may be similarly constructed and expressed repeatedly over the course of many months in the case of a long running show. One reason why intense emotion is largely proscribed in yoga is that it seems so unpredictable, but other systems suggest intense emotion may conform to patterns. One such pattern is that expression of emotion allows it to become something else, whereas inhibition either retains it or allows for a slower dispersal of it.

There is a concept espoused by the Japanese Noh theatre writer Zeami called *Jo-ha-kyu*. It means "beginning slowly" – "speed up" – "end swiftly" and he used it to express everything from the selection of works to be performed, the composition of each act in the play, and even the individual actions of an actor (Oida and Marshall 1997, 30–33). In other words, Zeami saw it as a universal concept for the patterns of movement in all things – from the cresting of a wave to the culmination of sex. One way to view emotional expression then, is to recognise that the flow of the emotion will burn itself out or transform into something else. The intense flare that emotion has as it burns most brightly is not easily sustained. The period that appears most dangerously volatile is short compared to the build-up. Yoga training is meant to facilitate a precise directing of energy to a specific goal which may be as simple as fiercely conveying energy to a part of the body to accomplish a feat of *āsana* or *vinyāsa* or as complex as channelling the energy of emotion as a fuel to surmount a challenge. As in the theatre context, where the channelling of emotion can be volatile, it would be important to recognise that the teacher (like the director) can call time out.

A third option, one that could be attributed to modern yoga, is to believe in the ability to deliberately change an unwanted emotion to a desirable one – anger to love, sadness to joy, or frustration to contentment. If Asma and Gabriel (2019) are correct, it is possible at the foundational level of sensory input, prior to the contextualisation accomplished by memory, and the application of the narrative lens of culture, that feelings are quite similar. At this foundational level, it seems possible that sensations can be interpreted in a variety of ways. An afficionado of tattooing may interpret the sensation of 'needling' as ecstatic rather than painful. The pleasure they feel (meaning) is a result of the contextualisation of their past experiences getting inked and the personal importance that the tattoo represents (cultural significance). However, pricking their finger with a sewing needle might produce a very different response. The question is whether they are simply creating a "heightened and individual interpretation of emotional response", or deliberately changing a negative emotion into a positive one. The latter seems improbable, simply because at the foundational level of sensory input, the reaction is not yet a response.

It has not yet, according to Asma and Gabriel (2019), been given full emotive meaning. If it were to be possible, it would require that one reframe the memories that assign primary meaning to the sensations. It may be that with spontaneous sensory input in the natural world, the process of contextualisation occurs too quickly to derail. But in a setting like the theatre or yoga, might one be able to anticipate sensation and channel it through the secondary and tertiary levels to produce a desired emotion?

From the perspective of yoga philosophy, one aims to free oneself of attachments, both past and present, to realise the nature of reality. Being able to stop the contextualisation and narration (conditioning agents akin to *saṃskāras* and *vāsanās*) may allow one to achieve a state of nonattachment. But this would appear to result in an absence of emotions rather than the good feelings that modern yoga desires. And, considering their important role in meaning making, how would a lack of emotional response change the nature of the practice experience? If emotions may serve as an intense fuel for yogic exploration, a practitioner will have to conceive of the contextualisation and narration phases more like an actor does – as malleable – and devise techniques to explore their pliancy.

## NOTES

1. This is a summary of part of Csikszentmihalyi's notion of the way in which emotions play a role in establishing and maintaining the state of 'flow'.
2. In the case of warfare, those who survive the battlefield together commonly tell of the bond shared by veterans. This is a special bond which cannot be understood by those who did not experience the intensity of battle.
3. Dialectical behaviour therapy (DBT) is a type of talking therapy. It is based on cognitive behavioural therapy (CBT), but it is specially adapted for people who feel emotions very intensely. The aim of DBT is to help one understand and accept their difficult feelings, learn skills to manage them, and accept the reality of their life and behaviours.
4. *Vinyāsa* is a method of physical yoga practice where one attempts to achieve continuous evenly paced movement linked with continuous and evenly paced breath. It seeks to explore the self and the nature of reality through a focus on sensory exploration.
5. According to Csikszentmihalyi a certain amount of challenge is needed to accomplish a state of 'flow'. As he states: "The best moments in our lives are not the passive, receptive, relaxing times ... The best moments usually occur if a person's body or mind is stretched to its limits in a voluntary effort to accomplish something difficult and worthwhile".
6. A ritual is stylised, repetitive behaviour performed for a purpose. In the process of ritual action meaning is interpreted symbolically. Rituals embody the beliefs of a group of people and if successful create a sense of continuity and belonging.
7. For a further analysis of the limitations on the understanding of the self, see "A Thing of Beauty" (Chapter 3 in this volume).

8. The meaning of bodily sensation is easily manipulated. It is not uncommon for modern teachers of yoga to define the meaning and impact of physical sensations for their students. Though this may effectively define the parameters of a student's practice experience, it also attenuates this same experience, limiting the possibility of what may arise through self-exploration. Presuppositions are the enemy of scientific exploration.

## REFERENCES

Asma, Stephen and Rami Gabriel. 2019. *The Emotional Mind: The Affective Roots of Culture and Cognition.* Cambridge, MA: Harvard University Press.

Csikszentmihalyi, Mihaly. 1990. *Flow: The Psychology of Optimal Experience.* New York, NY: Random House.

Damasio, Antonio. 2000. *The Feeling of What Happens: Body, Emotion and the Making of Consciousness.* London: Vintage.

Grosz, Stephen. 2014. *The Examined Life: How We Lose and Find Ourselves.* London: Vintage reprint Edition.

Hewitt, James. 1991. *The Complete Yoga Book: The Yoga of Breathing, Posture, and Meditation.* London: Rider.

Lewis, David, trans. *The Life of Teresa of Jesus* – (Teresa of Avila [1515–1582]). Ithaca: Cornell University Library, 2009.

Nevrin, Klas. 2008. "Empowerment and Using the Body in Modern Postural Yoga". In *Yoga in the Modern World,* edited by Mark Singleton and Jean Byrne, 113–139. New York and London: Routledge, 2008.

Oida, Yoshi and Lorna Marshall. 1997. *The Invisible Actor.* London: Methuen.

Rawson, Philip. 1973/1987. *Tantra: The Indian Cult of Ecstasy.* London: Thames and Hudson.

Sugarman, Anna. 2022. "Are Emotions Stored in Your Hips?" *Ekhart Yoga.* Accessed 2 April 2022. https://www.ekhartyoga.com/articles/practice/are-emotions-stored-in-the-hips.

*Yoga Sūtras of Patañjali* by Vivekānanda, Svāmi. 2012. Yogaville. VA: Integral Yoga Publications. Revised edition.

Chapter 3

# A Thing of Beauty

Benjamin Gillespie, writing in *PAJ: A Journal of Performance and Art* quotes David Byrne in his performance of *American Utopia*: "We're not fixed, our brains can change. Who we are thankfully extends beyond ourselves . . . to the connections between all of us" (Gillespie 2021). From a developmental perspective, our personalities become more or less defined, or bounded, by the organisation of neural pathways that occurs throughout the process of cognitive development. When you are born, you have multitudes of potential neural connections and the process of gradually reducing most of these is characteristic of aging and the development of personality. This development is a process of consolidation of habitual pathways that serves to functionally eliminate some neural options, rather than expand them – selectively limiting neural pathways to serve the conformity of one's sense of self. By eliminating some options and selecting others, we create an efficiency of neurological response at the expense of plasticity. We let go of what we don't need and keep the connections that are useful or relevant based on a version of who we believe we are. Personality, therefore, creates hidden constraints on our perceptual and intentional skills; constraints which define how we perceive and function in the world.

## THE LIMITS OF PERSONALITY

What if we could make ourselves so free of rigid conceptual boundaries of personality that we extend ourselves beyond such constraints and engage with that which is alien or 'Other'? One of yoga's ambitions

DOI: 10.4324/9781003471752-5

is to see the self as something that is not confined by the physical constraints of the mind/body. It strives to overcome the idea that the individual self (who our personality says we are) is separate from the 'Self' that is universal.[1] One method to accomplish this would be to acknowledge this rigid sense of who we are and *create* a more fluid and malleable sense of self, one that surmounts previously held beliefs and connects with that which we see as Other. To attempt this, yoga uses somatic techniques and the imagination to create new neurological connections that extend the limits of our habitual structures. Learning inversions (headstands, forearm balances, handstands, etc.) provides one common example of this process. Novice practitioners often observe inversions as something beyond their ability – they are *not* someone who can do a headstand – they believe they can't go upside-down and still relate to the world. The first experience of successful execution of a headstand is therefore accompanied by a feeling of rapture that is, in part, the realisation that they are now a person who *does* inversions. Such a shift in perception of self can open the door to other perceptual shifts, including those which connect to things that are beyond us. When we practice things that are physically challenging, we have the opportunity to gradually recreate ourselves by imagining possibilities and pursuing them. Cultivating this openness to other possibilities facilitates learning and each successive mastery (no matter how small) encourages greater openness – an openness which exceeds the physical accomplishment. When we have novel experiences or learn something new (e.g., to speak a language, to play an instrument, or to execute new postures or sequences), we create new neural pathways and, in embodiment terms, this results in a more fluid, less bounded, sense of self (Nevrin 2008, 125).[2]

In the opening monologue of his production, *American Utopia,* David Byrne suggests that this is precisely what is needed to fix, heal, and realign contemporary American Culture – "We create the fantasy of separateness" born out of our desire for individuation and sustain it based on our need to maintain a clearly defined and delineated sense of self. Byrne speaks of the necessity for empathy in a world which is currently characterised by strident and strongly held beliefs – a culture divided by solid lines marking distinct and competing worldviews. Byrne affirms the necessity of imagination in this endeavour, as it is a vehicle for unsettling the "fantasy of separateness", so that we might appreciate the reality of the connectedness between all things. Through this process of imagination, one might write or compose or paint to *create* new possibilities, rather than reflect on what already appears to exist. The creative process becomes a template for "getting out of ourselves" and positing a different reality (Byrne 2022).

## BLURRING THE BOUNDARIES

Yoga can be a creative process that frees us from the constraints of personality and then connects us to that which appears to be Other. Though the creative process is often rooted in experience, it can still challenge existing conceptual paradigms rather than reinforce or reiterate what we already believe. In addition to the developmental neurological processes, another possible barrier to expanding our experience comes from the way the modern yoga community is structured. The divisiveness and rancour seen in American society is mirrored, to some extent, within yogic institutions, where competition amongst orthodoxies and styles has led to a separation of traditions, each with their own sense of primal authenticity. Strident reductionism may appear in two varieties: those that simplify complex phenomena – answer complex philosophical questions with simple, or single variable solutions (e.g., meditation is the singular method to enlightenment) – and those that narrow the options for explanatory or observational frameworks (e.g., the self is foundational and immutable). Complex processes and phenomenon are reduced to simple procedures validated through history, lineage, or today, even science. In particular, the staunch belief in the primacy of ancient knowledge as the foundation of yogic philosophy and practice results in a muting of the possibilities for creative exploration. It presumes that the answers have already been discovered (even if this knowledge is unknown to most), and so, the focus of exploration and discovery is limited to reconfirming these truths.[3] In this environment, the procedures for achieving yogic goals risk becoming narrowly prescribed as do the rules for practice and discovery. In these circumstances, the opportunity for changing one's viewpoint, and thereby one's sense of self and others, is considerably restricted.

But what if our explorations could be untethered from the constraints of limited thinking and absolute rationality.[4] In yoga, the creative process may be used to illuminate the latent beauty of reality; to play with ideas rather than purport facts. *Vinyāsa*, like *āsana*, is the study of self and the study of reality, however, it is also the study of the ways in which we understand the self as it mingles with this reality. *Āsana* assumes a changeless reality (sought through efforts to achieve stillness) as it attempts to discover a changeless foundational Self.[5] *Vinyāsa* perceives reality as ever-changing and is premised on an appreciation of this ceaseless flow. In *āsana*, the constraints of personality are abandoned through the negation of self as a way to reveal reality. In *vinyāsa*, the acceptance of the flux and flow of the self and reality, renders these same constraints transitory.

## A THING OF BEAUTY IS A JOY FOREVER (KEATS 1818)

The notion of beauty is elusive. It can be understood as an ideal in the same way that "God" or "Love" have been in religion, but abstract or inexplicit concepts risk making us indifferent to beauty's experiential importance. By contrast, we might claim that beauty just isn't that interesting at all. Like appetite or thirst, it is simply the satiation of our aesthetic predilections and what more is there to discuss? You inhale the scent of a beautiful flower – and then? How long can one stay enraptured in the scent? Some claim they can stand in front of a painting for hours, letting it wash over them, but how much of that time is spent awaiting the next wave of stimulation or appreciation? The experience requires patience – the skill to stay engaged in inquiry waiting for novel stimuli to emerge. When we have the patience to direct our attention toward discovery, we develop an awareness of beauty. This helps us to understand the nature of reality. Through repetition and observation, novel stimuli are revealed which provide a motivation for continuing to explore even while doing the same thing over and over again. Elsewhere, we propose that contemporary yoga is an aesthetic philosophy (Clark and Greene 2022, *Teaching Contemporary Yoga*) – a toolbox of techniques for the sensual appreciation of reality (while earlier generations of yogis may have employed their techniques to achieve a complete negation of sensual engagement) (Eliade 1969, 66). There is no need to *understand* the concept of beauty in order to *experience* it. Waves of interest come from sensual stimulation and not from the appreciation of an abstract ideal. The acknowledgement of novel stimuli exposes the normal constraints of our personality and allows for the possibility of surpassing it to form new neural pathways.

One of the yoga-relevant connotations that beauty evokes is rapture. Enraptured before a sunset, or listening to great music, or viewing an exceptional piece of art, we are having the experience of beauty. Though some practitioners still seek ecstatic rapture through yoga (e.g., cosmic consciousness, enlightenment, or bliss), most practitioners spend relatively little time seeking these states let alone experiencing them. If yoga is pursued as an aid to a state of altered consciousness, something in the techniques must enable us to access it at will, without spoiling its wonder. No one needs to be trained to "see a sunset" but repeated exposure to a piece of music or a painting or a sculpture – or multiple sunsets – might make us blasé or inured to their beauty. Because yoga techniques involve considerable repetition, the trick is to find the ecstatic in the mundane.

For some practitioners, *prāṇāyāma* is boring, "It's just breathing, and I already know how to breathe". Meditation may be dull because "I'm just sitting!", and basic sun salutes or postures are uninteresting because

"I already know how to do this". There are also yoga practitioners who believe that the intense stimulation of extreme postures is necessary to sustain interest. Whether postures and movements are simple or extreme, repetitive or novel, grace is achieved when the appropriate amount of energy is expended in execution. In the experience of beauty, we acknowledge the engagement between our self and the one reality with which we all mingle. The appreciation of beauty cannot be forced (through extreme postures or other preferences); it is the result of a mingling that is energetically appropriate. Reality and the self are simply interesting and there is the potential to experience rapture in all things.

So, how might we dependably experience this beauty in the mundane? After all, a yoga practitioner might lose interest if they feel their questions have been adequately answered. This implies that novelty or *uncertainty* is interesting and that when one thinks they know it all, it is more likely to become dull. Yoga techniques, even if repetitive, become interesting if they dependably result in the experience of beauty. This is the feeling of connection to that which we perceive as Other; when new neural pathways are created and both consciousness and engagement are expanded and explored. David Byrne (2022) contends that contemporary culture suffers from a restriction of thought that fosters a rigid sense of self and an inability to perceive the complexity of reality. To create a less rigid sense of self, a yogi seeks to construe their experiences in a new way, one that does not preclude their predilections, but which allows them to see the novelty in everything. It is the continuous creation and expansion of new "pathways" which might enable a more profound connection with that which is Other, and which allows us to better see reality from an evolving perspective.

## IMPLICATIONS: THE FUTURE IS NOW

### The Role of the Imagination

People generally have a hard time seeing yoga as a creative endeavour. Without imaginative elements informing the practice, modern yoga seems ill-prepared to solve the kinds of problems that concern Byrne. There is a conservatism that supposes the only authentic yoga is comprised of ancient wisdom and questioning of this status quo and alteration of practice or philosophy is commonly met with accusations of appropriation. The assumption that there is a precise way to practice (discovered by the ancients and enforced through community, practice style, or orthodoxy standards) restricts the innovative ability of modern practitioners.

In Western cultures, there is a distinction made between the artist and the artisan. Craftmanship implies a high degree of skill, but it is something anyone can learn to do, and the crafts themselves, although admired for their execution and functionality, do not challenge conventional interpretation. An artisanal pottery plate is still a plate. Art on the other hand may be executed with similar skill, but in addition, it challenges its audience to reinterpret its creations in a new way. If we put the pottery plate in a plexiglass case in a museum, its aesthetics are appreciated differently. It is now not merely a "plate" but generates meaning through an exercise of the imagination – symbolic interpretation. This symbolic frame also promotes experimentation. Art and ritual are places where one is permitted to violate rules, question beliefs, and reimagine reality. Through this dynamic process, a culture's, or an individual's, beliefs are simultaneously challenged and reaffirmed, providing an opportunity for reflection on, and the amendment of, these beliefs.

In yoga, the self is traditionally meant to be realised without ego, judgement, or individuation, so the brash qualities of the artist would be largely unacceptable in a yogic innovator. Like the artisan's creations, the activities in a yoga class are both skilfully executed and viewed as principally utilitarian – this will "aid in digestion", "relieve stress", or "prepare you for splits". They are easily interpretable. Creative acts that may spawn imaginative and symbolic interpretation are largely absent because they are seen as either ego ridden or inauthentic. This lack of complex and variable symbolic interpretation leaves open the possibility for significant innovation in the future. The ritual context of the studio provides a safe space where one can challenge perceived wisdom, imagine other possibilities, and test theories that they might devise. It is a laboratory for discovery or innovation. Acknowledging and utilising the symbolic nature of yoga practice and the ritual context of the studio would certainly encourage creative acts of experimentation and bring practitioners closer to an understanding of the connectedness between all things.

## Being the Other

According to sociologist Fred Davis "breaking through" is a series of social strategies deployed by a stigmatised individual to change the way others (normals) perceive them, and thereby diminish the sense of difference. Davis described the mechanism of breaking through as "a redefinitional process in which the handicapped [here, stigmatized] person projects images, attitudes and concepts of self which encourage the normal to identify with him [sic]". In this way, the stigmatised individual "disavows the deviancy latent in this status" and "the 'normal' comes to normalise (i.e., view as more like himself [sic]) those aspects of the other which at first connoted deviance" (Davis 1961, 120–122). For this to occur, the stigmatised individual and the other must engage in significant (and sometimes prolonged) contact where new identities may be negotiated, ideally to the point where the stigmatised is seen as a person rather than a set of preconceived traits. This kind of knowing – one that renders the Other as fully human – is needed if we are to see past the narrow frame of understanding that maintains Byrne's "illusion of separateness" (Byrne 2022). The opportunity for deep connection is already available through the application of *vinyāsa* yoga philosophy and techniques for sensual engagement. But how might the studio become a place where this engagement deliberately occurs?

The idea that one plays a role in a yoga class may appear offensive to some. After all, a yoga class is a place where ethics and honesty are paramount virtues and there is a dishonesty found in not-being-yourself. To suggest that the yoga class is really some sort of cosplay featuring people in tights sounds like a Marvel Superheroes meets Fitness Trends Convention. Is the yoga class really an appropriate forum for escapism? Regardless, there are roles aplenty essayed during class. For some, the roles of the yoga studio are liberating. For the intemperate, it might be an opportunity to plausibly entertain what it would be like to behave virtuously. For a conformist, it might be the chance to find a rebellious maverick within. The trope of the "best self" or "true self" can be conceived, explored, and defined in a safe environment. The studio is a place where people can try out looking like a yogi. What that means is unique (or should be) to each individual. Some might decide to sit or stand with a much straighter spine than they would normally as part of their definition of what they might look like. They might claim to be interested in veganism. They might earnestly attempt to make unusual shapes with their body and sit in contemplation when their day job requires the muscular attitude of a steelworker. A shy person can feel exonerated from portraying themselves as they would ordinarily and become more socially outgoing.

It is not just the student who plays a role in the studio. The teacher too, assumes a certain demeanour that is different from who they portray in workaday life. Deliberately or not, they model themselves as avatars of yoga for their students. It is where their definition of yoga is given lived public form, but with the safety net of an audience already pre-disposed to liking the result (simply because it is yogic). The life of yoga is taken from the conceptual and given lived form in the interactions of the studio. Participants at cosplay events claim it gives them confidence, a sense of belonging, and an outlet for their creativity. Parallel claims could be made for yoga.

But too often, the roles are cliché ridden. Like in the world of cosplay, one cliché is that yoga will be particularly good to you if you are good looking. Consequently, 22-year-old yoga teacher impersonators or weekend workshop shamans have their own You Tube channels where they can spout a version of ancient wisdom and modern health tips. This is not because of their knowledge, though they most likely have at least some certification, but because they execute a sufficiently convincing and pleasing rendition of the character of attractive yoga teacher or far-out shaman. There is, arguably, an important difference between cosplay characterisation and the role one assumes in a yoga context. The context of cosplay is that this is overtly dressing up in tribute – the character and the impersonator are distinct. In theory, dressing up in cosplay does not imply consent to be wholly treated as the character would be treated if they existed in real life. Characterisation in yoga does not make this caveat – what is presented in a yoga context is what one is inviting others to treat as real. So, in one sense, the stakes at risk are high – the role assumed is the one you wish to be taken for; not merely a fan's tribute. It could be that this high risk has resulted in the relatively tame and virtually archetypical choices made for yoga studio role playing. Yet, this is an area where particularly adventurous strides could be taken. As long as everyone understands that this is role play, the ritual situation of studio and class gives more scope for subtlety in character interpretation. How might one essay the role of an ancient mountain *ṛṣi* arriving at the modern-day studio? What might the Goddess Kali wear to class? How does an authentic modern yogi behave? And how might they behave when they depart? Cosplay is created in imitation. We are advocating the creation of character through imagination and integration of the creators aims in life. David Byrne (2022) asks us to consider how we might invent new ways of being in the world that stretch us beyond our previous versions of self and that allow us to empathise with the views of others. Assuming the characteristics of others – taking on the physical mind set of other ways of thinking and being in the world – is one of the ways this might be accomplished. Imagination is an under-utilised ability that, when applied, can allow the yoga practitioner to break through to fully engage with the Other and allow for new ways of understanding reality.

## NOTES

1. *Āsana* and *vinyāsa* are two major techniques for practicing physical yoga. In *āsana,* postures are held for a period of time in an effort to approximate absolute stillness and lack of sensory information from the outside world, and thereby actualise a foundational self which does not change. This foundational or essential self is found by turning one's attention inward once the body is

able to achieve the unchanging stillness found in pure consciousness (*puruṣa*). *Vinyāsa* by contrast seeks a flow of continuous, even movement, approximating the flow of time. It seeks to understand the nature of the self as it interacts with the Other, both of which are in constant change. The focus of *vinyāsa* is outward, savoring sensory information to understand the nature of reality and the self as it moves within it.

2. Commenting on the work of Smith (2002) and others.
3. The problem of 'confirmation bias' is certainly common in the sciences as well. Great care should be taken to minimise both 'observer's bias' and confirmation bias whenever experimentation and exploration are conceived and carried out.
4. Rationality functions reliably with what is possible given the constraints of data driven parameters regardless of their actual truth. Reason, on the other hand, requires that one draw conclusions and allow for possibilities that are contingent. They ask questions like, "what if we could . . .?" rather than disregard the conditions found in potentiality.
5. The Foundational or Essential Self is thought to be equivalent with the unchanging and eternal Pure Consciousness that makes up all that is known as *puruṣa*.

## REFERENCES

Byrne, David. 2022. *American Utopia* (Broadway, NYC performance) August 3, 2022.

Clark, Edward and Laurie A. Greene. 2022. *Teaching Contemporary Yoga: Physical Philosophy and Critical Issues.* London: Routledge.

Davis, Fred. 1961. "Deviance Disavowal: The Management of Strained Interaction by the Visibly Handicapped". *Social Problems* 9 (2): 120–132. https://doi.org/10.2307/799007.

Eliade, Mircea. 1969. *Yoga: Immortality and Freedom, Second Edition.* Translated by Willard R. Trask. Princeton: Princeton University Press.

Gillespie, Benjamin. 2021. "David Byrne and the Utopian Imagination". *PAJ: A Journal of Performance and Art* 43 (3): 7–18. muse.jhu.edu/article/805405.

Keats, John. 1818. "A Poetic Romance". In *Endymion.* London: Taylor and Hessey.

Nevrin, Klas. 2008. "Empowerment and Using the Body in Modern Postural Yoga". In *Yoga in the Modern World,* edited by Mark Singleton and Jean Byrne, 119–139. London: Routledge.

Smith, Mary Lynn. "Moving Self: The Thread Which Bridges Dance and Theatre". *Research in Dance Education* 3 (2): 123–141.

SECTION II

# THE SOCIAL WORLD

Chapter 4

# What Really Matters

For many, modern yoga simply provides a path to fitness or relaxation, but for some, it offers an opportunity for liminal experience[1] as well as a place of belonging. In contemporary Western culture, rites of passage marking life transitions may have been lost, or at least, significantly transformed – recreated and redirected into liminal experiences that allow the individual to redefine their identity and their place within the larger society. Modern yoga has become firmly entrenched in Western popular culture and is arguably the fastest growing wellness practice of the last few decades. Between 2018 and 2023, despite the Covid-19 pandemic (or maybe because of it), yoga practitioners in the United States increased by over 50%. In 2023, worldwide, approximately 300 million people were regularly practicing yoga (Yogindra 2023). What can account for the popularity of this practice and its continued growth in both Western and Eastern milieus? Modern yogic rituals centre around the body and aim to clarify and contextualise mundane experience by providing techniques to define individual identity and establish a meaningful place within a community. For many practitioners today, absent traditional rituals and rites of passage that would help to clearly define social roles and identity, yoga functions as a ritual of transformation that privileges individual spirit.

## RITES OF PASSAGE: NAVIGATING SOCIAL AND PERSONAL TRANSFORMATION

Rites of passage, a concept popularised by Arnold van Gennep, mark the passage of a person through the life cycle, from one stage to another over

DOI: 10.4324/9781003471752-7

time, and from one role or social position to another, thus integrating social and cultural experiences with one's biological reality. This process is inherently about understanding one's "self" and its place within the larger social and even cosmic reality. Though van Gennep concentrates on universal rites that designate transitions between life stages (e.g., birth, initiation, adulthood, marriage, death), he acknowledges that there are many kinds of rites that function to meet the specific needs of modern societies. For each rite of passage, van Gennep identified three stages – "rites of separation from a previous world (preliminal rites), those executed during the transitional stage (liminal or threshold rites), and the ceremonies of incorporation into the new world (postliminal rites)" (van Gennep 1977, 21).

In nonindustrial (traditional) societies, rites of passage are typically uniform and uniformly applied. Members of nonindustrial cultures have clear expectations about their future roles and the status changes that will accompany them. Their purpose is more or less clear as is their pathway to this purpose. In modern industrial societies, people are free to seek secular or religious rites that serve to create a sense of self that connects them to others in meaningful social groupings. In short, one is able to choose the social affiliations and social identity one finds most meaningful and reflective of their perception of the self they wish to realise. But this freedom of choice is accompanied by challenges unique to industrial societies – high levels of structural differentiation,[2] that often result in feelings of isolation, identified by Emile Durkheim as *anomie* (Durkheim 1893). For Durkheim, *anomie* is a state of "normlessness" – the lack of social cohesion and solidarity that often accompanies rapid social change and the increasing division of labour. Concomitant with modernity, an increasing division of labour weakens one's sense of identification with the wider community and thereby, among other things, weakens constraints on human behaviour.

Thomas Merton later redefined Durkheim's concept of *anomie* to refer to a:

> . . . de-institutionalization of means brought about by an imbalance that exists between society's *cultural goals* and institutional means whereby the goals are over-emphasized. The state of anomie thus characterizes modern societies as a whole, a condition that is brought about by the fact that, for example, the American dream – a two car garage, a home in the suburbs, a comfortable living – is widespread even when the means to achieve it are not within reach. Anomie is a social condition, not an attribute of individuals.
>
> (Delflem 2018, 147)

Both Durkheim and Merton were interested in criminality and other antisocial and nonnormative behaviours (like suicide) as ways to negotiate or resolve this inherent incongruity. But one might also consider *anomie* as a generalised motivator of social behaviour to combat the cognitive dissonance which enables it. Absent a clear or viable path to overemphasised cultural goals, individuals may look to more socially acceptable accommodations to resolve the dissociative feelings.

## THE SHIFTS IN CULTURAL GOALS

Durkheim and Merton framed cultural goals within the context of Marxism or the social institutions of Functionalism.[3] We would argue, along with others on the political left and the right (Fine and Love 1999, 285–299), that cultural goals have shifted since the 1960s in particular, and then again in the 1990s. Though financial gain remains a prime motivator for behaviour, wealth is no longer enough to achieve success. New cultural goals have come to the fore, especially for those who see themselves in opposition to what they believe are stagnant and unenlightened mainstream cultural values. As historians William Fine and Nancy Love state in their review of the literature on the Sixties:

> Even the most oppositional and seemingly subversive features of sixties movements are viewed more as reflections of society than as challenges to it. Cultural innovations are selectively incorporated by a generally supportive populace. Activists who sought an impossible revolution or a leap into utopia help bring about changes far different from those they intended . . . radical politics becomes a quest for personal freedom and authentic identity . . . A paradigm of progress emerges in which culture becomes an expression of agency, and material concerns yield to questions of meaning and identity.
> (Fine and Love 1999, 286)

These new or expanded cultural goals create an emphasis on personal empowerment. Internationally, cultural goals trend toward aspects of self-improvement, whether this be vocational, relational, or spiritual. Once radical aims enter the realm of popular culture, they lose their revolutionary character. The 1960s radical call for equality of all beings has been translated into inclusivity and nonjudgement. The lofty quest for self-realisation becomes a striving for personal happiness and "living one's best life". The expansiveness of cosmic consciousness is replaced by a cultivation of intuition and empathy. Concomitantly, the commune, which afforded the opportunity to "drop out", has been replaced by paid membership in institutions (like the yoga studio) that emphasise community and belonging. And the goal of "overcoming death" has been translated to the achievement of optimal health. As one practitioner describes:

> To me, personally, [yoga] is a way of staying in the moment without worrying about things outside of class. It has given[sic] me more empathy for others

> by connecting me to an amazing community. It has healed me in so many ways, I really feel like a better person. I may not be a yogi in the old sense of the word – according to the east – but to me, the definition of yoga is peace.

Religious scholar Andrea Jain argues that these changes in meaning are the result of the commodification of yoga in the context of neoliberal[4] capitalism. She contends that "Personal growth", "self-care", and "transformation" are all tropes in the narrative of the "spiritual identity", presented as countercultural or "alternative", but to the contrary, are "mainstream and sometimes even conservative and nationalistic". Though spiritual seekers may acknowledge the obsession with "athleisure apparel" that push socially conscious merchandise, or "therapeutically-focused applications" that emphasise healing the person rather than the broken system, their critiques are mere gestures – amounting to tag lines on tee shirts (Jain 2020). Whether one agrees with Jain's critical critique or not, suffice to say that modern yoga has lost much of both its countercultural ambition and its radical transformational agenda.

## YOGA AS A MODERN RITE OF PASSAGE

In the face of shifting or shifted cultural goals, the rise in the popularity of modern yoga, in particular physical yoga, may be partially explained by the alignment created between a dedicated practice and the progress toward these goals. Practice is made more potent, especially when enacted as a ritual in the context of group studio classes. During rituals of practice, the world and the human body are intricately intertwined and mutually engaged in exploring the transpersonal. The studio provides a venue for this exploration, and the community there can act as a powerful supportive structure. Participant observation[5] and interviews collected by the authors over a ten-year period[6] confirm the importance of the studio as a ritual venue and the shifting cultural goals with which it is aligned.

Studio practice can easily be analysed as a ritual – both as a rite of passage and as a rite of intensification.[7] A yoga practice has many ritualised elements and follows the structure of ritual enactment. Special clothing is required for practice, and one is asked to remove their shoes and socks in the practice environment as an act of reverence. Special jewellery with spiritual significance may be worn and placed beside one's practice space or may be utilised during practice. Clothing may be traditional and uniform (as in Kundalini Yoga, for example) or more revealing than would be acceptable in other venues – men may practice with bare chests and women wear form fitting clothing or may even practice in a sports bra.

Religious historian Klas Nevrin (2008) has thoroughly analysed the importance of the environment for practitioners' understanding of yoga and their practice experience. The studio may be adorned with devotional iconography from Eastern traditions and an altar may be situated in the front of the room on which ritual items are placed. These items are symbolic of the principles on which the studio is founded and are evocative of each student's spiritual pursuits. Props particular to practice (e.g., blocks, blankets, bolsters, and straps) must be utilised in particular ways and cared for as respected objects. In the Iyengar Yoga system, for example, there are precise and prescribed ways to fold blankets, arrange blocks, and cinch straps used during practice. Practice occurs on a special yoga mat which is kept clean and serves to demarcate each individual's ritual space. Intrusions into this space are met with reproach. There may be incense burning, dimmed lights or candles, and soft music playing. A ritual language may be used, be it special yoga jargon, or Sanskrit (itself considered a sacred language) which is also chanted or sung in *māntras*. These *māntras*, like spells, are performatives – they accomplish what they profess as they are invoked, even if those present are unaware of their meaning. The sounds themselves are believed to have alchemical properties. As Nevrin states:

> . . . similar practices may be interpreted and experienced differently, depending on the context in which they are performed . . . stylistic differences are not only a matter of holding different beliefs but include the way in which a practitioner will *feel* in a particular practice environment. Many practitioners will, for example, emphasize the ways in which a particular practice environment might induce a sense of stillness or calm; a sense of belonging; an energized motivation; or a "spiritual atmosphere." . . . The stylistic differences will be important for whether the practitioner feels at home, or whether he or she has a sense of the atmosphere being right for them.
>
> (Nevrin 2008, 121)

In sum, Nevrin illustrates how the environment shapes and contextualises experiences that arise within the practice session. The importance of contextual features in forming experience is also emphasised by philosopher Alphonso Lingis. In his provocative analysis, *The Imperative*, he argues that not only is our thought governed by an imperative (as Kant had maintained) but, rather, our sensual, sensing, perceiving, and emotional life is continually regulated by imperatives generated from the world around us. He shows that there are directives in the natural world and in our interactions with others that govern our thought and behaviour – the Other guides our experiences (Lingis 1998). We are not simply entering a neutral space when we enter the studio or *yogaśālā*. We are entering a ritual context that shapes our experiences.

The practice itself, of course, is also ritualised – it is a highly structured routine. As we have described elsewhere (Clark and Greene 2022, 45–69), whether sequences are fixed or variable, a yoga class follows a structure that correlates with the three stages of ritual progression – separation, transition (liminal), [re]incorporation – outlined by van Gennep. Movements are stylised, repetitive, and performed for a specific purpose, one that requires a symbolic, interpretive frame. Talismans (fetishes, or magical objects) may be used to intensify one's experience or assist in transformation. When entering a practice session, one leaves the mundane order of their everyday lives and enters the liminal phase of transition. This may happen at various times for individual practitioners but, for most, it has occurred by the time they take off their shoes and place their mat on the floor of the studio. As one practitioner related:

> At the beginning of each class, [the teacher] asks us to turn our thoughts inward. She encourages us to check in . . . what kind of state we are in bodily and mentally. We spend a few seconds reflecting on what brought us to practice and what we hope to gain from it.

And another describes the process of separation at her studio:

> The lights were dimmed, the atmosphere was inviting, and I slowly started to forget about the small things that had been bothering me. I unrolled my yoga mat and sat with observant eyes. The instructor introduced herself to the new participants who had not practiced the week prior and gave everyone a brief overview of the class we would be participating in that night. The class started, and I felt myself begin to relax.

The majority of the class, led by the teacher acting as the ritual operator, is liminal – practitioners are taken through a series of challenges in which their attention is drawn to various somatic and evocative stimuli. The final posture, *śavāsana*, begins the reincorporation stage as students assume the posture of a corpse, only to be reborn transformed. This transformation is typically sealed with the collective chanting of *Oṃ*, and the practitioner then exits the studio to return to their ordinary lives.

> As the class began the yoga instructor handed out angel cards to each of us and told us not to look at them until the end of our class . . . The instructor went on to explain that the angel cards are meant to help with guidance in someone's life. She said yoga is meant to be a guide for one to be fulfilled physically and spiritually; the practice is meant to push our mind and body and have them work with each other instead of against each other. I enjoyed her comparison and how to combine physical activity and spiritual activity . . . When the class began, and again when it ended, the teacher started by having the class take three big deep breaths in, and as we exhale, we say *om*. I thought it was a good spiritual way to cleanse the mind and to center

> one's mind to do the yoga practice and then later to take what was learned during the yoga practice throughout a person's day.

During a practice session, students are instructed to interpret shapes and movements in symbolic terms, either through leading instructions (e.g., open your heart in this posture) or through more indirect means. One way indirection may be accomplished is through the telling of a parable at the beginning or during the class session, or both. One practitioner tells of her practice the day after the massacre at a concert in Las Vegas:

> I took a class the day after the shooting in Las Vegas . . . All of the students entered class with heavy hearts. Melissa decided to have us all dedicate our practice to the survivors and victims of that horrible night. I dedicated each pose I did to the individuals who are in the hospital and for the ones who passed away. It was so powerful, I cried for them.

Controlled breathing is another aspect of ritualised behaviour that characterises yoga practice. Though there are various methods of breathing, the most common breath used in physical practice (*ujjayi*) is both metered and audible. Breathing is maintained for the duration of practice, and, ideally, only ends at the (re)incorporation stage (*śavāsana*). Brain scientists have suggested that metered breathing may have important biochemical implications. "Paced breathing increases release of prolactin and oxytocin . . . which can promote feelings of calmness and social bonding" (Torner, Toschi, Clapp, and Neumann 2002, 1381–1389). In the context of group practice, the sound of another's breath becomes an intimate exchange that promotes a feeling of community. As one practitioner notes:

> We sync up our breathing and say our *ohms* together, which has a calming affect over us all. Although I just started attending yoga a month ago, I feel as if I made new friends and have another place I 'belong' too. The whole class is bonding as one to expel the old air out to make way for the new air and to clear out our minds.

And as another notes, the synchronisation of breath is akin to a prayer – making the practice sacred:

> Sometimes you can hear the soft breaths of those around you as well as your own breath . . . These external sensations all come together to form a place of relaxation. They allow you to feel the rhythm and match your flow with everyone else, like a moving "prayer". When you can achieve this, you are able to let go of things that may have impacted you throughout the day and fully turn your attention to what is happening right there in the now. A place that allows me to reach this state is a place that becomes "sacred".

*Śavāsana* (corpse pose) is important, as "analyses of modern rites of passage (e.g., Outward Bound, certification programs, black belt bestowal) have found the impact was lessened by the missing [re]incorporation phase" (Cushing 1998, 7–12). Another practitioner describes her favourite class:

> The instructor I go to . . . Heidi, likes having the light slightly dim, lights aromatic candles, has a little Buddha, wakes you up from corpse pose with the yoga bowl . . . and uses music to set the mood. She also sets the tone at the beginning of our practice by speaking of what to focus on for the day. For example, when I went to her class last Saturday she spoke about the feeling of conceit and how you have to let that go and be humble. She also usually relates the postures we are doing with the message of the day. Another thing she does is at the end of the practice, when we are resting in corpse pose, she will add a drop of essential [oil] to your resting palm I guess as a reminder to take the message with you. I feel like she gives her practice a more mystical tone. Without that, I don't think I'd feel so different after.

The importance of the ritual aspect of a studio practice cannot be overstated. It is why practitioners suggest that yoga is not simply about the body, but a practice that is about the mind and the spirit as well. It is a search for something more than the mundane concerns of fitness and health – although these will also figure in practice – as body centric notions of health and fitness act as an entry point into alterations of consciousness and transformational pursuits.

## YOGA AND THE CONNOISSEURS OF CONSCIOUSNESS

Yoga is different from many other physical pursuits in that it claims to surpass simple concerns about fitness of the physical body. Connoisseurs of consciousness are those who practice these "higher pursuits". In yoga, connoisseurship comes in one of two general varieties: those that discriminate through an eliminative process versus those that discriminate by learning through experience. The eliminative process presumes that there is an irreducible state of consciousness (that may be referred to as "pure consciousness") that can be obtained through the rigorous recognition and discarding of all input from the material world. In Saṃkhyā philosophy, the Sanskrit term applied to this state or experience is *puruṣa*. This fundamental state is posited as a reality wholly separate from materiality. The process of learning through exposure still makes use of discriminative discernment, but its difference from the eliminative process is that it accumulates insight through observation and appreciation of difference. It is not the either/or of the eliminative discernment of material versus pure consciousness, but rather, the appreciation of a multiplicity of differences (derived from a world external to the individual or from an inwardly sensed realm). The connoisseurs of consciousness seek to discriminate through what cursorily appears to be two diametrically opposed processes that also appear to be equally conflicted in their broad definitions of consciousness. One defines consciousness as unchanging as well as indestructible and in no way to be confused with the individual, the personal, or the characteristic. It is undifferentiated. The other considers consciousness to be multiple, variable, and approached through its constructions and interpretations of the material world. This kind of consciousness might be felt as emotion or perceived as a process that constructs meaning.

There are also two kinds of physical yoga techniques used to explore consciousness – stillness and continuous movement. Through stillness or movement rituals, one strives to negate the body's influence (*āsana*), and thereby the "self" or celebrate the body in an active engagement with the "Other" (*vinyāsa*). In either case, the world, and the human body, are intricately intertwined and mutually engaged in exploring the transpersonal. For the eliminative, because it is foundational and unchanging, transformation is only pertinent in the moment one realises the state (pure consciousness) – the state does not (and cannot) transform. The energy that gives form to an inanimate thing, like a rock, is the same energy that holds an animate body together – and has nothing to do with individual human consciousness except insofar as it is a consistent and ongoing phenomenon of energy that a human being takes part in for the duration of its human existence. The opinionless "knowing" of this might be said to be illumined consciousness. Traditionally, the yoga techniques that set out to achieve the transformation to this "knowingness" involved trying to find disengagement from the material world and from individual personality. This self-negation might consist of assuming postures (*āsanas*) and remaining still or shutting the eyes to remove the visual distraction of the material world. Practitioners would then look inwardly to find the state of irreducible energy. They also might hold their breath for extended periods of time. Their efforts were meant to bring about a ritual "death" to living in the material realm so that they might be "reborn" to a way of truly experiencing the actuality of existence without the transitory, and possibly illusory, perceptions through which humans construe the world. The connoisseur sought to know that Self and Reality are ultimately the same thing – everlasting, unchanging, and indestructible.

The second kind of connoisseur is a modern phenomenon. They engage in an appreciation of the *moment* rather than the eternal; in the transitory and unique rather than the unchanging and indestructible; the multiple rather than the unitary. The yoga techniques utilised here may require an outward engagement with the world coupled with deep sensorial observation. This outward engagement involves movement into the world rather than retreat from it and, in many ways, is a celebration of the individual "self" as an expression of the universal "Self". This connoisseur seeks to know the self and its relationship to all that is Other – it sees the self and the world as everchanging and interdependent.

## CONSCIOUSNESS: OUTWARD FORMS AND INNER STATES

Defining consciousness is notoriously difficult. From the perspective of yoga philosophy, consciousness is ephemeral yet fundamental. Contemporary practitioners, however, largely understand consciousness as knowable. This is their modern interpretation of *haṭha* yoga traditions wherein, through bodily refinement (rather than philosophical pursuit), one may achieve a refined mental state. Modern practice has implicitly accepted that outer form is meant to correspond to an inner state.[8] The authenticity of the mind, or soul, or invisible realm of spirit is revealed to be the same as the visible outer form of the body. Internal stress is to be found in external tension. Inner calm is expressed in outer ease. A congruence between these inner/outer or invisible/visible manifestations of consciousness are understood by the practitioners to provide windows on something larger than simple human consciousness – they reveal something about the nature of being. The practitioner becomes the metaphor for what reality is – a perfect piece of 'being' as expressed through a human body. Consciousness allows for one to imagine, invent, and project idealised states in which alternate realities are created or explored for the purpose of transformation. In contemporary yoga, consciousness allows for the interpretation of being through the human form.

The meaning and use of the body in practice has also been altered. Whereas the ancient yogis sought to overcome the body to achieve transcendence, modern practitioners aim to categorically accept their bodies to find a community and their place within it. Body positivity, inclusivity, and nonjudgement are central to the ethos of modern practitioners. Transcendence is today more about the cultivation of ethical pursuits than energetic transformation. Whereas ancient yogis sought to move and refine energy at various levels of their bodily existence for alchemical purposes, modern practitioners have come to pursue energy primarily as a means to refine their ability to intuit and empathise on a transpersonal level. The strength of feelings induced by the experience of practice – deep stretching, synchronised breathing, rigorous movement, intense heat – create states of consciousness which are interpreted as "spiritual". The manipulation of the body is not wholly mundane – the shapes of the postures have limited utility – they are certainly not the most direct way to achieve physical ends like building strength or flexibility. Understanding postures as symbols allows for the interpretation of the body as a vehicle for spiritual investigation. The community has become the conduit for this spiritual experience. Consciousness is invisible, yet tangible in that one may have a sensorial experience of it while engaging with the selves of others. Modern practitioners' understanding of consciousness is practical. It is the way that their self and the selves they are engaged with coexist. Therefore, the studio is the place where heightened consciousness can be pursued through the shared ethos within a community.

## TRANSFORMATION: TRAUMA AND HEALING AS MODERN IMPERATIVES

Embodiment theorists contend that consciousness is formed phenomenologically – created through the body's lived experience – and so the world and the sense of "self" are emergent phenomena in an ongoing "becoming" (Merleau-Ponty 1962). Merleau-Ponty emphasised the body as the primary site of knowing the world, a corrective to the long philosophical tradition that positioned consciousness in the mind". Merleau-Ponty maintained that the perceiving body and its perceived world could not be disentangled from each other as Cartesian duality contends. In modern practice, connoisseurship, and consciousness itself, are rooted in the material world and are embodied. To be spiritually attuned for the average practitioner is to be "living one's best life", having "manifested one's reality" in a "healed body" purged of "trauma". The yoga practitioners interviewed frequently described their experiences in yoga as a "journey", rather than an attainment of a specific goal. One practitioner describes finding yoga while searching for something akin to religion:

> Yoga has been another milestone in my spiritual journey. Even as a young child, I was always worried about praying to God or being a good child of God. I always wanted my godparents to take me to church on Sundays and prayed every morning and every night. As I grew older I decided that the catholic religion is not the right one for me, so when it comes to religion I feel kind of homeless. I have tried to visit different churches and even got baptized as a Mormon . . . and still am dissatisfied. I realize now that I am so obsessed with doing the right thing or believing in the right church that I could not really enjoy my spirituality. When I started doing yoga, I started to maybe think I did not need a religion and maybe yoga could be my religion.

Not all journeys are pilgrimages rooted in overt religious or spiritual pursuits. Just as frequently, "journey" references a personal quest for fulfilment outside the bounds of religious worship. A long-time practitioner, for example, describes her first yoga class:

> The teacher sat at the front of the room and told us a story of how her yoga journey through the years helps cure her self-esteem issues. This sparked something in me. I had been to therapy, but I felt lost. I didn't have a way to reintegrate myself into my social circle. My own journey had just begun and since my divorce, I felt like regaining self-worth would be the focus of my own struggle.

Still others speak of the value of yoga as they begin their transition to adulthood. A male college freshman talked at length about how he got into yoga to improve his soccer skills and prevent injury, but instead found a way to transition from his high school self to his college self:

> Overall, I would say that my yoga journey was a successful one. I mean, my flexibility is better, and I feel strong out on the field. Mostly it gave me a reason to stay here on the weekends and not go home to party with my high school friends . . . I don't need to go home, I'm done with that. It's mostly friends going nowhere. Hopefully my yoga journey will continue beyond this semester as there is still so much to discover both about the practice and about myself.

The designation of practice as a "journey" indicates that the process of practice is one of discovery. This discovery is accomplished by manipulating the body in ways that result in a transformation of perception. Consciousness is altered through the actions of embodied discovery.

Within the emergent ritual yogic experiences observed here, embodied threats to the social order are commonly evoked (e.g., trauma (past), toxicity (present), and anxiety (future)) that may then be expressed in ways that are transformative and cathartic. Trauma, whether physical, emotional or both is understood as a basic human condition that clarifies the goal of human spiritual transformation – release of the trauma (and possibly trauma from past lives) in order to find the transformative state of enlightenment. Enlightenment has been redefined as the purging of past traumas so that one might actualise their true self through healing. Examples of these sentiments abound in testimonies. As one practitioner states of the impact of heat on his body:

> Hot yoga has been even more of a life-changing experience in this way; the heat in the room, and the heat created in me as a practitioner, successfully burned away impurities. The teacher began class by asking us to find something burdensome that we came to class with and led us through class while continually reminding us to let this thing go and release it as we move to release our sweat and toxins. The entire session was physically and mentally very cleansing and healing, especially with certain situations that are

occurring in my life right now. I felt like all that trauma, the stuff I held without knowing burned away.

Another speaks of the purging of "toxins" both physical and ethereal:

> . . . as we were doing the practice the teacher said phrases such as "move into downward dog to release the toxins in your legs". In my experience, there has been a lot of talk of cleansing the body by removing the toxins. Also, the teacher told us a story of how her yoga journey helps cure depression. Although not a physical ailment, statements such as this claim to heal the body from the inside out. In all of my yoga classes . . . the teacher would say something about how yoga can be a healing practice. For example, in the experience stated above, the teacher communicated to us how the body can be used as medicine in an encouraging way. I have found that when I can picture in my mind the invisible toxins releasing me it helps push me to challenge myself at the practice. Almost always the teacher communicates yoga as medicine in explaining how it cures aches and pains or mental issues that a person may be dealing with but not even be aware of.

Modern practitioners' transformation is commonly focused on healing from physical or emotional trauma. Practice results in a catharsis, emphasising the importance of emotional response in the transformational process and the ritual nature of the experience of practice. As we have written elsewhere in this volume (see "Minding the Body", Chapter 1), emotional response originates in the body as a "postural attitude" – the tonicity needed in the body to ready oneself to express an emotion – a necessary substratum of action that is a prerequisite for movement and therefore emotion (Jacobson 1970, 34). Emotional response, and the changes in consciousness associated with it, are therefore also phenomenologically rooted.

Many practitioners also spoke of trauma as a somatic reality. Pain in the hips, for example, might be indicative of relationship trauma and one's heart can "close" due to physical or emotional trauma and need to be "opened" through physical practice. Trauma is generally recognised as universal and is stored in the body as "toxins" which when released, have simultaneous physical, mental, and spiritual effect. As one practitioner notes:

> In order to truly heal, one must let go of the concept of control. One must let go of the desire to be perfect, the need for something to fill the void, and the need to escape.

> Yoga will heal. When *tapas* are created in practice, and heat ignites and boils away impurities from within, emotional and mental healing will likely follow – as long as the ego lets go of any of its expectations, and the yogi lets go of his or her concept of control. . . . Especially with my experience of yoga, I felt a lot more limber and the constant sweating made me feel happier and

> lighter on my feet afterwards . . .When I leave the class, I feel the endorphins from my practice and that only made me excited to come back the next chance I could to *surrender* and *release* even more so I can find my self and my purpose in this world (authors' italics).

Apparently, the release of toxins (established through past traumas) is perceived to be accomplished through the process of physical surrender and release. The practitioner sees it as a physical and emotional process that results in a shift in consciousness; a consciousness that is moving toward their self-actualisation. Embodied physical release invokes a similar release internally. The necessity for physical yielding is based on the assumed correspondence between internal and external states. For consciousness of self to be accurately observed, one "surrenders" to abandon both the physical and thought patterns (established through experience and cultural metaphor) that might mask or override its unencumbered flow. The physical surrender and release are meant to allow consciousness, likewise, to be released – freed of the logical strictures that bind rationality and inhibit exploration beyond what is already known.

## THE ROLE OF COMMUNITY IN CONSCIOUSNESS

One manifestation of this belief is in the increasingly common practice of 'trauma bonding'. Trauma bonding occurs when both authority and relationships of trust are built through the sharing of trauma stories. Trauma bonding has become a common technique in yoga teaching. Teachers may gather their students at the beginning of class to take an inventory of injuries – physical, emotional, and psychological – in an ostensible effort to best lead their students to a positive transformative experience. This affirmation of students' trauma experiences (which are embodied) is first played out in what linguist Deborah Tannen and others denote as "troubles talk" (Tannen 2007) – when people (mostly women) share stories of emotional pain. The fact that communication might be feminised in the contemporary yoga community should come as no surprise, since the vast majority of yoga practitioners today are women.[9] When trauma bonding occurs in a public or communal context, the healing potential becomes communal as well.

Trauma bonding is commonly used as a way to forge relationships within the studio setting. Trauma bonding is the intensification of feelings of connection brought about through the sharing of highly personal stories of trauma. The more intense these stories of trauma, the more potential they hold, and speaking the stories aloud can result in a "groupfeel" that encourages empathy for the teller. But why is trauma considered an acceptable emotional response and encouraged as a tool for transformation when anger is not? The reasons for the acceptability of the expression of trauma and not anger may have to do with the way that trauma stories uphold the power relationships within any social context. While public expression of anger may be seen as inappropriately aggressive – a way for the speaker to increase their relative power – expressions of trauma place the speaker in a position of self-deprecation. When a teacher initiates trauma bonding by telling their personal stories of struggle, or loss, or failure, they are ostensibly lowering themselves to the level of the student in an attempt to bond with them. It is, intentional or not, a manipulation of their students meant to create an illusion of closeness through sameness.

Yoga practice has transitioned from a solitary enterprise to one that is strengthened by, and legitimised in, intentional communities where real (and often inchoate) embodied threats are addressed. In the past, the role of the traditional *guru* was to obliterate the ego of the disciple (*śiṣya*) through a series of formal rituals that transitioned the disciple from novice (*bābā*) through protracted stages of initiation. This was a lengthy process, a lifetime practice, and way of life. Today however, the teacher is more likely tasked with facilitating a student's healing – a healing that is both personal and transpersonal, and never completed. Essential to this modern process is the community itself, which serves as a partner in the exploration of the boundaries of consciousness. It does so by being a place where the practitioner is free to explore their consciousness through their imperfect bodies. As one practitioner states:

> In my mind, "community" means a group of people with common interests or habits, who feel a sense of solidarity towards each other, or towards the group as a whole. Having a sense of community within your practice space is key for successful practice. When I am practicing, I want to feel comfortable, safe, and accepted. If I am practicing in a space where I don't even feel comfortable breathing aloud, odds are that I will not allow myself to engage in the practice mentally or physically, therefore not benefiting from my practice in the way that I should. Though the practice of yoga is a very personal journey, the community within your practice space can dictate the direction and the impact of your journey.

There must be trust in the community for one to feel safe when engaging in exploration of the physical body and consciousness. Likewise, the community provides support for these explorations since all are perceived as engaged in a mutual and similar process. As a young woman fairly new to yoga commented:

> Our sense of community provides for the studio an environment where we can just do our best . . . without feeling judged . . . Overall, we seem to be

> reasonably engaged with each other and supportive in a space where we can all practice and gain whatever it is that we need for our own bodies and minds. Having a sense of community in our studio is beyond important. It makes our class feel whole, like we are one person.

This feeling of belonging is important. For those who crave it, the *yogaśālā* is home to an intentional community, one that replaces more traditional groupings – kinship, religious affiliation, political association, guild – that once clearly defined one's sense of self and life's purpose. This community is all accepting – it is a place of "nonjudgement" and is "mutually supportive". The intensity of this acceptance, and the support and encouragement that it provides, is integral to the success of the rituals enacted there. As other research has also shown, the context of the ritual is as important as the ritual itself.[10] The studio becomes a liminal space supported by the community. This support is also crucial for the healing that must necessarily take place for consciousness to be explored and eventually evolved. As practitioners have expressed, the difficult "journey" to overcome everyday (or more deep-seated) trauma that takes place in the studio is possible only because of the mutual support of the community who are all "there for a common purpose" and act as "inspiration for one another".

## WHY CONNOISSEURSHIP MATTERS

Unlike early Western countercultural experiments in yoga, modern yoga in its popularised form, is largely domesticated and makes yoga now suitable and accessible to everyone (Jain 2014). It is no longer couched within the confines of Eastern religion, but rather in the secular, physical, and spiritual body of the individual practitioner as they seek self-realisation. In the past, yogis aimed for the loftiest goals. They sought total annihilation and an abandonment of society and their own ego identities, or an interaction with the Other in which they were at once self and god (Self). Today, connoisseurs of consciousness look to others in their chosen community to guide them through this exploration, an exploration which is embodied, yet interpreted as ephemeral. "Enlightenment" if it does occur, will be found through interpersonal ritual interactions, in which a community can easily and quickly create powerful traditions that facilitate transformation for its members. Sometimes these rituals are created instantly, as when the teacher polls students as to "what they want to work on", attesting to the dynamic nature of studio interactions. The success of these rituals is experienced simultaneously on a physical and ephemeral level – intense bodily experiences are interpreted as transformations of consciousness. These transformations are perceived as "evolutions" of consciousness or "higher vibrational frequencies" which allow the seasoned yogi to "intuit things that others cannot hope to perceive". Evidence of this thinking can be found in the *QAnon* movement and other countercultural responses to both Trumpism and the Covid-19 pandemic. In both instances, many in the yoga community aligned themselves fiercely with conspiratorial beliefs. When questioned about their positions, yogis responded by claiming to "know things others can't see", and hoping others would "wake up already". They believed that, through practice, their consciousness has been elevated (they "vibrate at a higher frequency"); their intuition refined (they "just know things").

Some might argue that these changes have largely come about because of the diminishment or lack of rites of passage and other traditions that successfully transition individuals from one life stage to another. As Durkheim and Merton have attested, structural differentiation has caused social dissociation which has resulted in the loss of clear roles in social groupings. With the loss of designated roles comes the subsequent loss of rituals to mark and make these transitions. Rituals were also meant to educate as well as facilitate transition so that new roles might be embodied and executed with confidence. In their absence, the studio community has taken over the role of the traditional shaman or priest.[11] Absent clear direction through formal rituals, studio members assist in the navigation of generalised anxiety which accompanies the search for meaning and one's purpose in life. Almost every practitioner interviewed spoke about their anxiety – sometimes expressed as "stress" – and the healing which yoga provided. Regardless of the understanding of consciousness or the technique used to evolve it, yoga provides a venue for this exploration – a chance, through belonging, to find meaning and a place where they can assuage the anxiety that accompanies modern life.

## IMPLICATIONS: THE FUTURE IS NOW

As Klas Nevrin (2008) has suggested, the environment in which one practices is not a neutral space – it generates stimuli that manage our experience and helps to make meaning. The studio is a recent innovation in yoga as is group practice with formal classes. The ancient yogis had specific rules regarding the parameters of their solitary practice space, which were followed to ensure success. As the *Haṭha Yoga Pradīpikā* describes:

> The yogi should practice hatha yoga in a small room, situated in a solitary place, being 4 cubits, and free from stones, fire, water, disturbances of all kinds, and in a country where justice is properly administered, where good people live, and where food can be obtained easily and plentifully.

> The room should have a small door, be free from holes, hollows, neither too high nor too low, well plastered with cow-dung and free from dirt, filth, and insects. On its outside there should be bowers, raised platform (*chabutra*), a well, and a compound. These characteristics as a room for Hatha Yogis have been described by adepts in the practice of Hatha.
>
> (Sinh 1997, 1:12–13)

And from the *Śiva Saṃhitā*, a further recognition of the importance of the practice space: "Let the Yogi go to a beautiful and pleasant place of retirement or a cell, assume the posture *padmāsana*, and sitting on a seat (made of kusa grass) begin to practice the regulation of breath" (Vasu 1996, 3:20). The *Bhagavad Gītā* (6:11) describes the use of antelope skin and kusa grass.

Jacqueline Hargreaves and Jason Birch point to the importance of the selection of a surface for practice as they are summarised in the *Puraścaraṇacandrikā* – a compilation on the preliminary rites (*puraścaraṇa*) for mantra recitation (Hargreaves and Birch 2016, webpage). Before teaching postures (*āsana*), Devendrāśrama includes a number of verses on the types of mat (also called *āsana*) on which the practitioner should sit:

> Hear of the Āsana [mats] which have been prescribed by sages. One should know that a tiger's skin brings success in all things; a deer skin is for mastery over [one's] location; a mat of cloth destroys illness; one made of cane increases prosperity; a silk [mat] is nourishing [and] a woollen one alleviates suffering.
>
> In [performing] rituals that harm enemies, [one should use] a black [mat] and in rituals that subjugate [others], etc., a red one. In pacifying rituals, a white [mat] is prescribed and in all [other tantric] rituals, a variegated one. In rites that paralyse [others], an elephant's skin and in death-dealing rites, a buffalo's skin. [Alternatively,] in rites that expel [enemies], a ewe's skin and in rites of subjugation, a rhinoceros' skin. In rites that cause dissension, a jackal's hide is prescribed and in pacifying rites, a cow's hide.
>
> When repeating a universal mantra, [sitting] on a bamboo mat [causes] poverty [and sitting] on a wooden one, misfortune. [Sitting] on the earth causes suffering and on stone, disease. [Sitting] on a straw mat destroys one's reputation and [sitting] on [one made of] twigs causes mental distraction. And [sitting] on [a seat made of] bricks results in anxiety.
>
> An initiated householder should never sit on a spotted black antelope skin. An ascetic, a forest dweller, a celibate (brahmacarī) and one who has taken the ritual bath [to mark the end of Brahmacarya] should sit on a completely square [mat] made of Kuśa grass, antelope skin or cotton, raised up one or two hands or four finger-breaths [from the ground].
>
> (Hargreaves and Birch 2016, webpage)

Considering the ways that the practice environment is said to manage the experience of practice, one can imagine that *haṭha* yogis experienced practice quite differently. In fact, one could argue that the practice space is key in creating practitioners' belief that yoga is different – it is "more than exercise" – it has a "spiritual" aspect as well.

Aspects of the practice space whether they be mats, iconography, music, incense, or even the very characteristics of the space itself are all attributed meaning specific to the ritual context. In conjunction with the ritual nature of the practice, there is a real opportunity for deeply meaningful experience. How might future yogis best manipulate the parameters of the practice space in a way that reflects contemporary culture to help ensure the outcomes they seek?

The newest and most rapidly expanding venue for practice is online. Some practices are interactive in this space (e.g., Zoom) and some are recorded (e.g., YouTube). Since the Covid-19 pandemic, increasing numbers of students have chosen to continue taking classes online (because they are easy to access and convenient) but at a cost. Online classes create challenges for both the teacher and the remote participants who will each be in a different environment. This environment may lack ritual meaning (e.g., one's living room) to manage the depth of experience. In addition, teachers (as ritual operators) lack control of the ritual environment and must rely solely on their verbal cues and the visuals of their practice space to assist students in exploration. Modern yogis seeking "more than exercise" may want to create (or already have) ritual contexts of their own or designate ritual spaces within mundane ones (e.g., a yoga and meditation room) to enhance their explorations. The growth of online classes coupled with the mainstreaming of yoga practice in gyms, senior centres, and the like has also resulted in the necessary denuding of the ritual context. This has altered the meaning of yoga from an ascetic discipline to a fitness and wellness regimen. Yoga was traditionally a solitary pursuit. Wandering mendicants left their homes and villages to practice without the constraints of family, community, and other social obligations. They required this untethering, they believed, in order to fully dedicate themselves to exploring the ineffable. Today, community is, to a great extent, the arbiter and supporter of yogic explorations. The growing popularity of both online classes and healthful practice may account, in part, for the ubiquitous popularity of teacher trainings today because they provide a meaningful context for practice and situate an individual firmly within a community of belonging. The community has become the most important influence on the nature and meaning of experience and it is no wonder studios promote their "shared community" in marketing.

Traditional societies had clearly articulated stages of life that were marked by rituals – ensuring, through meaningful rites of passage that individuals would be well integrated into the social order. They would understand the social responsibilities and rights associated with each status as well as the process entailed in achieving the next stage. The traditional stages in Hinduism are *Brahmacharya* (student life), *Gṛhastha* (household life), *Vānaprastha* (retired life), and *Sannayāsa* (the life of the renunciate – yogi). The final stage was a sort of dis-integration from material society into the order of solitary yogis. Today, in contrast, yogis frame their social evolution as a "journey" without a series of set stages. How does maintaining the concept of "journey" effect the outcomes of practice and the reason one practices to begin with, and are there other ways of imagining stages of life that fit modern yogic pursuits? In the absence of formalised rituals and clear roles and stages by which they are acquired, modern yogis will continue to depend on others to frame their understanding of themselves and their relationship to reality.

One such example is the prevalence of women who begin their yoga practice in midlife. For many, they come to yoga as a way to figure out their place in society – they have aged and are no longer valued in the way they were in their youth. They may have raised their children, been married and divorced, feel dissatisfied with their career, and generally feel a loss of power in a culture where aging women become invisible. Yoga is a way to find themselves and their place and role within a community which does not judge them.

The ancient *haṭha* yogis felt one should devote themselves to practice before age and infirmity sets in, and similarly today, the strong physical practices are mostly for the young. But, in the Hindu tradition, in ancient times, the elderly might seek a wholly spiritual life as wandering mendicants – *sannyāsins* – rejecting their name, their family, and their former place in society – devoutly seeking, at the end of their lives, a way to pass out of human existence into whatever may follow with equanimity. Modern yoga for the elderly, rather than focussing on the inevitable life transition from living creature to corpse, attempts to provide elderly practitioners with a taste of how good it feels to move – provides the delight of feeling movement and breath even if merely executed while sitting in a chair. This is not to belittle the palpable delight that is experienced by the elderly who may be reminded of what it was to be alive with youthfulness and to experience their old age in a way that they are the best that they can be. Such experiences *could* conceivably have a role in accepting death with equanimity, but they are not cast as such. It is here that the resolutely upbeat and happy voiced yoga instructor may appear at their most infantilising as they take the elderly through simple movements with "Good job!" encouragements to those who, in previous times, might have been revered as repositories of wisdom. While death meditations (contemplations of the disintegration of the body) have long been a part of yogic practice, it is not something that is widely integrated into Western yoga for the elderly. In the past, the wisdom of the elders showed the way to a satisfactory end of the "journey" – death. Today, the concept of a journey in yoga is that it lacks a predictable trajectory or end. Absent a formal structure, the journey risks becoming a vain attempt to capture or recapture health or youthfulness rather than consciously prepare for one's death.

## NOTES

1. Liminal experiences provide a means for novel experience, the redefinition of one's worldview, and the opportunity for ecstatic experience. Within these experiences, the rules for mundane existence are suspended, including the individual's current social status and role, making the outcome of the ritual uncertain. Exploration is possible, but not without risk – the danger lies in the lack of certainty that results from entering a liminal space.
2. Structural differentiation may be defined as the tendency for human societies to evolve toward increased differentiation, in which institutions become increasingly specialised in the functions they perform. This differentiation may result in the loss of function for traditional institutions and render traditional roles obsolete or cause a loss in their agency.
3. Functionalism, in social sciences, is a theory based on the premise that all aspects of a society – institutions, roles, norms, etc. – serve a purpose and that all are indispensable for the long-term survival of the society.
4. Neoliberalism is a political philosophy that emphasises the individual's personal responsibility for their social reality rather than the inequality created through stratified social institutions.
5. Participant observation is an anthropological technique for investigation. It involves both observing and participating in the research site. It is the principal embedded and embodied investigative method.
6. The methodology for this research combined participant observation with open-ended interviews. Both authors teach yoga as trainers and guest teachers in studios throughout Europe, the United States, Asia, and Mexico. Laurie Greene also teaches an academic yoga course in which students keep journals reflecting on their practice experiences. These journals were also used as ethnographic data. Direct interviews were conducted with individual studio owners, and with groups of practitioners who attend studio classes regularly.
7. A rite of intensification is a ritual in which the group, rather than the individual is transitioned to a new stage together.
8. This concept is found in various source materials on *haṭha* yoga. For example, the *Haṭha Yoga Pradīpikā* states that when the body is motionless, so is the mind.
9. Traditionally, yoga was almost exclusively a male pursuit.
10. This is particularly apparent in studies of the placebo and nocebo effect.
11. There are those in the yoga community that identify as shamans. Shamanism is becoming increasingly popular in yoga culture.

## REFERENCES

Clark, Edward and Laurie A. Greene. 2022. *Teaching Contemporary Yoga: Physical Philosophy and Critical Issues*. New York and London: Routledge.

Cushing, Pamela J. 1998. "Competing the Cycle of Transformation: Lessons from the Rites of Passage Model". *Pathways: The Ontario Journal of Experiential Education* 9 (5): 7–12.

Deflem, Mathieu. 2018. "Anomie, Strain, and Opportunity Structure: Robert K. Merton's Paradigm of Deviant Behavior". In *The Handbook of the History and Philosophy of Criminology*, edited by Ruth A. Triplett, 140–155. Malden, MA: Wiley-Blackwell, 2018.
Durkheim, Émile. 1893. *The Division of Labour in Society*. Universitè Presses France.
Fine, William F. and Nancy S. Love. 1999. "Review of Fighting for the Sixties: Political Movements and Cultural Change, by Paul Berman, James J. Farrell, Thomas Frank, Todd Gitlin, Arthur Marwick, Doug Rossinow, and Julie Stephens". *Polity* 32 (2): 285–299. https://doi.org/10.2307/3235287.
Hargreaves, Jaqueline and Jason Birch. 2016. "The Religiosity of the Yoga Mat". *Luminescent*. Accessed 22 April 2024. https://www.theluminescent.org/2016/04/the-religiosity-of-yoga-mat.html.
Jacobson, Edmund. 1970. *Modern Treatment of Tense Patients*. Springfield, IL: Charles C. Thomas.
Jain, Andrea. 2014. *Selling Yoga: From Counterculture to Pop Culture*. Oxford: Oxford University Press.
Jain, Andrea. 2020. *Peace, Love, Yoga: The Politics of Global Spirituality*. Oxford: Oxford University Press.
Lingis, Alphonso. 1998. *The Imperative*. Bloomington: Indiana University Press.
Merleau-Ponty, Maurice. 1962. *The Phenomenology of Perception*, translated by Colin Smith. London: Routledge, 1962.
Nevrin, Klas. 2008. "Empowerment and Using the Body in Modern Postural Yoga". In *Yoga in the Modern World: Contemporary Perspectives*, edited by Mark Singleton and Jean Byrne, 119–139. New York: Routledge.
Sinh, Pancham, trans. 1997. *The Hatha Yoga Pradipika*, 5th edition. New Delhi: Munshiram Manoharlal Publishers, 1997.
Tannen, Deborah. 2007. *You Just Don't Understand Me*. New York: William Morrow Paperbacks.
*The Baghdad Gita*, trans. by WJ Johnson. 1994. Oxford: Oxford University Press.
Torner, Luz, Nicola Toschi, Gabriel Nava, Carmen Clapp, and Inga D. Neumann. 2002. "Increased Hypothalamic Expression of Prolactin in Lactation: Involvement in Behavioural and Neuroendocrine Stress Responses". *European Journal of Neuroscience* 15 (8): 1381–1389.
van Gennep, Arnold. 1977. *The Rites of Passage*. Translated by Monika B Vizedom and Gabrielle L. Caffee (Paperback Reprint ed.). New York and London: Routledge Library Editions Anthropology and Ethnography. Hove, East Sussex, UK: Psychology Press.
Vasu, Rai Babdur Srisa Chandra, trans. 1996. *The Siva Samhita*. New Delhi: Munshiram Manoharlal Publishers.
Yoginidra, JR. 2023. *Yoga Earth*. "50 Blissful Yoga Statistics for 2023". Accessed 18 October 2023. https://yogaearth.com/yoga-research/yoga-statistics/.

Chapter 5

# When Credentialing Doesn't Matter

## THE UNIVERSE OF SPIRITUAL ENTREPRENEURSHIP

In the wellness industry, 'spiritual entrepreneurs'[1] often subscribe to creative theories to explain the principles and efficacy of their work – explanations that may defy scientific demonstration. Through their "offerings", these practitioners attract a clientele who are led to believe they are purchasing something more valuable than a mere product. Nebulous jargon is used to enhance the value of their services and support the efficacy of their practices. "Life changing", "energy empowerment", "manifestation", "the future you", "raise your vibration", "lower astral forces", and "coherence healing" are just a few such examples. These practitioners seek a clientele who consider themselves in need of psychological or physical therapy founded on energy-based principles. Like the career path of yoga teacher, the vocation of spiritual entrepreneur is both new and enjoying increasing popularity. There are many types of spiritual entrepreneurs, including yoga teachers, who regard their profession as a way to help others. Are these spiritual entrepreneurs qualified to administer to vulnerable people?

Spiritual entrepreneurs may believe that yoga, for example, is so unquestionably good for you that it is always beneficial. Though their experience as a yoga practitioner or teacher may be limited, they attest to their "love" of yoga (and other allied practices); a love based on the positive impact it has had on their own lives. This love becomes the foundation of self-credentialing and can render formal training or depth of study unnecessary. While their knowledge could potentially deepen, most often, absent a motivation for further study, the dedication is transient – transferring

DOI: 10.4324/9781003471752-8

instead to the next big spiritual thing (e.g., sound healer, numerologist, shaman). By choosing to offer a wide range of services, the entrepreneurial yoga teacher opts for breadth of offerings over the depth of knowledge that comes with a lifetime of dedication to a discipline.

What makes this vocation so seductive and the people that follow this path so popular? Perhaps it is because people see spiritual entrepreneurs as trailblazers in a hip counterculture community that they would also like to be a part of – being "their best selves" and "living their best lives". They might imagine becoming a trailblazer themselves, and so escape the mundane demands of their current careers. As part of the entrepreneurial marketing strategy, clients may be told they are special, that they have been selected to succeed, and that they too can be virtuous by choosing to dedicate themselves to helping people.

This notion of specialness is important to spiritual entrepreneurs. They may see themselves as privy to information unavailable to the general public. This, they believe, is due to "the work" – what they have done to achieve a superior level of spiritual evolution. They may conflate intuition, having read a book, or completing a weekend workshop with having done the work necessary for this special status. Their status is often justified by valorising so-called ancient knowledge and practices in opposition to Western ones (that are deemed tainted). This presumes that superior knowledge and spiritual insight were well known to the ancients yet, are now hidden from most in Western culture. In many ways, the rejection of Western culture is a rejection of modernity. The rejection of science, and the scientific method in particular, is necessary since much of what they choose to market, if subject to rigorous testing, would fail to be supported.[2]

## LIMINALITY, COMMUNITY, AND CULTS

So how might one further explain the popularity of spiritual entrepreneurs and their services as it applies to yoga? Coined by Arnold van Gennep in his work *Rites of Passage* (1977 [1909]), the term liminality was meant to describe a potentially transformative state – a "space/time/experience" – that exists between mundane experiences of reality. At its most dramatic, it facilitates an irreversible transition from one state of being to another (e.g., marriage, adulthood, graduation). Within this "space", status is suspended, and experiences are governed and interpreted by rules which are distinct from everyday reality and specific to that state. Van Gennep used the concept of liminality to describe why ritual experiences are so powerful and inherently unpredictable. Within these experiences, participants conditionally accept an alternate definition of their being, beliefs, and practices which may not make sense or be acceptable in everyday contexts. Upon exiting the liminal state at the conclusion of the ritual, participants are reincorporated into everyday reality, albeit altered by the experience obtained within the liminal state.

A yoga studio may be viewed as a liminal space as it is both physically circumscribed and the rules of mundane reality are suspended. The interpretation and meaning of actions (e.g., postures, breathing, and movements) behaviours (e.g., chanting, removing shoes, the use of a mat), and symbols (e.g., iconography, language, important texts) are specific to the ritual context of the studio and its members. What goes on in the studio is different from what goes on outside of it – it is a different reality that functions as a transitory state between the workaday and the spiritual realm. An individual yogi is meant to return to the mundane world altered, rather than to remain within the "studio reality" because liminality functions as a temporary condition. When someone enters an *āśrama* or a retreat centre, this liminal state becomes protracted and can be increasingly transformative, and disengagement and reincorporation may become more difficult. In an *āśrama* in particular, the community defines and enforces the boundaries of liminality. For successful incorporation into its specific reality, the *āśrama* community relies on people's desire to belong and find meaning.

In the case of cults, ritual operators are aware of the nature of the ritual process, but ideally, the participants are largely unaware of how intoxicating and powerfully transformative the ritual experience can be. Because of this, cult leaders and cult communities may convince participants that the liminal reality is actually *more* real than their everyday lives. This is possible because the community claims to have special knowledge that outsiders lack. Operators may manipulate participants in dramatic ways. There is a difference between cult leaders and some spiritual entrepreneurs, but this may only be a matter of degree. The belief in healing in the spiritual and wellness communities, for example, is often based on faith rather than on empirical evidence of its efficacy. Most of the impact of yoga as a healing modality is similar to the placebo effect (Smith, et.al. 2022). AJ Brown observes:

> When applied appropriately, yoga is the most eloquent of all placebos. It provides experiences and ideas that encourage a healing response. The benefits cannot readily be measured by scientific means and yet the subjective and anecdotal evidence of its effectiveness is more than can be stifled. Of course, yoga practice is quite diverse and, depending on which class you go to . . . it can just as easily become another culturally-induced nocebo that further disables us.
>
> (Brown 2014)

The placebo effect lies in the positive expectations it produces that derive from the larger context in which treatment is administered. Placebos require liminal conditions in order to express their greatest impact. The hospital is a ritual setting where individuals take on special roles relative to their status. These roles (be it doctor, nurse, janitor, or patient) are marked by symbols that indicate the individual's status and identity. For example, while in the hospital receiving treatment, a patient relinquishes their everyday status (and the rights and responsibilities associated with it – e.g., lawyer, father, athlete, even doctor) temporarily for the duration of their treatment and their everyday behaviour is both highly regulated and ritualised. They eat when and what they are specially provided, they wear a hospital gown rather than their own clothing, they are monitored and required to follow all the rules associated with in-patient treatment. They may only leave this status when they are formally discharged by the attending physician (Parsons 1951, Murphy 1987).[3] This period of liminality is maintained through the ritualisation of everyday behaviours, and it is precisely these behaviours and the ritual context in which they occur that enhance the effectiveness of the treatment received. As is noted in a blog post from the Harvard Medical School summarising placebo researcher Ted Kaptchuk:

> . . . [P]lacebos are not all about releasing brainpower. You also need the ritual of treatment. "When you look at these studies that compare drugs with placebos, there is the entire environmental and ritual factor at work", says Kaptchuk. "You have to go to a clinic at certain times and be examined by medical professionals in white coats. You receive all kinds of exotic pills and undergo strange procedures. All this can have a profound impact on how the body perceives symptoms because you feel you are getting attention and care".
>
> (Harvard Medical School Blog 2022)

It is possible that the ritual is more powerful than the placebo itself. This is significant because it points to the immense power of ritual to transform people, their thinking, and their experiences. For all we know, it is the ritual that accounts for the effect of the placebo rather than the "medicine" administered. The community (e.g., medical, yoga studio, reiki, etc.) controls the context and circumstances that make the ritual possible and give it specific meaning. It is easy to underestimate the potential power that communities wield through ritual action. In cases where a highly esteemed spiritual entrepreneur or other community leader acts as the ritual operator, this may be more profound. The spiritual entrepreneur uses the community's strongly shared values and beliefs to both substantiate their healing practices and manipulate their clientele – for good or for ill. In the case of cults, the spiritual leader may create the community and the worldview to which it subscribes. This places them in the position of being more than a "healer", for they are also the creator, the all-knowing, and the arbiter of all that is true.

## CREATIVE DECEPTIONS: ARTISTS AND SWINDLERS

There is a difference between the spiritual entrepreneur's creative use of imagination and that used by the artist with their audience. The artist asks the audience to suspend everyday beliefs so that viewers might entertain their creative vision. Everyone involved understands that this experience of art is imaginative and not the same as reality – it is liminal[4] and functions as a filter through which reality may be interpreted. For many wellness practitioners and their clients, this shared premise of conditionality is absent. The more strongly a conviction is felt, the more those who tend to rely on their *intuition* assume it to be true. Clients are led to believe that the creative concepts and claims of the practitioner are wholly factual rather than imaginative. The depth of feeling that accompanies certainty of belief or faith (either by the practitioner or client) can result in a culture where "knowledge" is intuited, rather than discovered through experimentation or formal educational institutions. The need for such beliefs is driven by the desire for certainty and the status that accompanies the perception of one's superior knowledge.[5]

In the contemporary yoga community, an interpretation of intense feelings about things not fully known can be understood as enlightened insight and may help explain why intuition is so highly valued. In *The Intuition Tool Kit*, Australian researcher Joel Pearson (2024) defines intuition as a tapping into one's interoception – an access to the unconscious through physical movement. Physical movement, he contends, is a highly accurate form of perception. The eyes, for example, can easily be tricked through an optical illusion, but when one moves one's hand into the field of illusion, the illusion vanishes. Movement, unlike vision, will not fall for the deception. Further support for the primacy of the body as a tool of perception is found in the accuracy of what we perceive to be intuitive responses. When we are in a heightened adrenaline state, we are likely to confuse the adrenalised feeling for intuition. According to Pearson, intuition is particularly untrustworthy in situations of heightened emotion. Arousal misattribution is the tendency to attribute strong feeling within our bodies to feelings for others. We may, for example, erroneously believe we are in love when a date at the movies is accompanied by strong, physically palpable, emotions. We misinterpret where the romantic feelings come from and transfer them from the film to the person we are with. Intuition is highly prized as an outcome of modern yoga practice; a skill that is akin the alchemical powers (*siddhis*) said to have been acquired by ancient practitioners as they advanced toward enlightenment.

But, according to Pearson and others, intuition is neither a sign of enlightened consciousness nor a dependable measure of the perception of reality. It is more akin to a kind of transference. We evaluate and interpret our bodily responses and experience them as a "knowing", whether accurate or not (Pearson 2024). In social interactions, the transfer of emotions can also colour and transform our own and others' consciousness. Strong feelings may give the expression of consciousness the appearance of authenticity. The more we *feel* something, the more we, and those who we interact with, also *believe* it to be true. Lying is a particularly telling and interesting human phenomenon for it illustrates how untrustworthy emotions can be – a convincing liar takes advantage of the gullibility of their audience by compellingly providing sensory information that the audience expects or hopes to observe.

Though intuition may be untrustworthy, there are advantages to trusting one's feelings which may account, in part, for the success the wellness industry enjoys. When a practitioner relies on their intuition, they do so through empathic interaction and respond to their client as an individual with a novel set of experiences which requires a unique approach to healing. In Western medicine, practitioners must follow set protocols uniformly when treating specific conditions – treatment options are curtailed by both scientific findings and public health or insurance institutions. Ironically, the latitude that wellness practitioners enjoy, and which bring them success, could be threatened by the acquisition of licensure through formal accreditation.

## THE NECESSITY FOR HEALING

Common to wellness practitioners is the importance of healing. According to the wellness community, virtually all people are in need of healing, whether it be physical, psychological, or spiritual and, therefore, require their services. Examples of this trope for the universal need for healing can be found in a variety of publications and is espoused by a multitude of practitioners. From the publication *Yoga Glo*:

> Whether it's physical or emotional, most of us have experienced some kind of pain at one point in our lives. We are all different, so we all experience pain differently and cope with that pain in different ways. Some hide and suppress it, *avoiding the healing process that we all need to go through in order to move on* [emphasis the authors'], while others decide that they no longer want their pain controlling their lives so they confront it. If you are having trouble healing or don't know how to heal, practicing yoga is great way to being [sic] the healing process.
>
> (*Yoga Glo* Blog 2014)

Aside from the need for healing, another point often made is the universality of suffering itself. Shannon Sexton writes in *Yoga Journal* that suffering is experienced everywhere in the same way:

> "Whether we're suffering from relationship trauma or low-back pain it wears on our consciousness in a similar way [quoting Tiffany Cruikshank]." Step into any yoga studio around the world and you'll likely find that many people in the room came to yoga because they needed to heal in some way.
> (Sexton 2014)

To lay claim to their role as healers, wellness practitioners often distance themselves from the world of fitness and exercise. As Trina Campbell states:

> What makes us different is that we are not trying to promote exercise, we promote healing. While doing a headstand is cool, that is not our main goal. We want to make a difference in our clients and help them find and maintain their personal space of physical, mental, and spiritual healing.
> (Swart 2021)

Because they believe that everyone needs to be healed, practitioners have little to offer people who feel fundamentally healthy. The clientele they seek are those who are suffering. Once clients believe that they are healing, they will trust the spiritual entrepreneurs and heed their advice.

The popularity of the wellness industry has led many Western medical practitioners and health services to incorporate holistic health practices into their services in an attempt to increase *their* client base. An example comes from this traditional addiction rehabilitation facility:

> Yoga, an ancient system that balances the mind, body and spirit, helps to maintain physical health while centering the ever-wandering mind. Here at Delray Center for Healing, patients in our care can utilize yoga as a part of their mental health treatment plan. This provides the opportunity to experience the many mental health benefits that yoga has to offer.
> (Delray Center For Healing)

Here, the authenticity of ancient knowledge is invoked as a way to express the cutting-edge services offered by this facility. This presumes that the people providing these services have a deep knowledge of ancient practices and have seen their efficacy – they must be applying these practices as the ancients did. Facilities often use yoga as a way to attract clients without providing any specific proof of the benefits attributable to the practice as a therapy. There are people in the wellness community who are well trained and quite knowledgeable, however, many who incorporate holistic practices, including yoga (as spiritual entrepreneurs or in medical facilities), are not. They are simply using these services as a marketing tool. The clients themselves have only limited knowledge of authentic ancient practices, although they do desire the gentleness they believe accompanies these energy-based therapies (and holistic medicine in general) when compared to Western healing regimens.

The appearance of authenticity is crucial for spiritual entrepreneurs. They may align themselves with indigenous, ancient, natural, or time-tested healing traditions, and combine them in novel ways. Innovation or novel combination are not necessarily appropriation, although it may genuinely be mistaken for it. Appropriation is when source material from a culture is unacknowledged, misrepresented for one's own gain, or dismissed, so that a practice becomes more accessible to those outside of the culture of origin. It denudes the tradition through simplification, without acknowledgement. For example, they might claim that what they do is incorporate common elements of "shamanic practice" found among indigenous people world-wide in cultures they have never encountered (a violation of ethical standards in anthropology and academic study). Those elements are stripped of their specific cultural content so as to render them accessible to contemporary Western spiritual seekers. As shamanic practices have become quite popular in the world of holistic healing (*ayahuasca* as a noteworthy example) of which yoga is a part, it is wise to question the intention of these practices and from where they arise. In a desire to move away from what are perceived as impersonal and unnatural Western medical practices, clients may seek what they believe are more authentic, natural, and gentle treatment regimens – ones that they believe will benefit them physically, mentally, and spiritually. But in making these practices accessible for their clients, spiritual entrepreneurs may be selling appropriative offerings that are little like the authentic ancient practices from which they originate.

## DOCTORS OF MINISTRY

Despite the dubious association of wellness offerings with ancient practices, a variety of spiritual entrepreneurs and their services continue to enjoy popularity. This explains why some titles are so frequently invoked as spiritual vocations – Coach, Healer, Entrepreneur, Trainer, Worker, Shaman, and even Minister or Doctor, but not Lama, Monk, or Priest. The latter are perceived to require a more formal disciplinary structure; one that removes one from a life lived to its fullest. If the former terms appear overused or inappropriately applied, it may be because they are unregulated and are not subject to standard licensure or institutional definition (Goldacre 2006).[6] Some titles (minister, for instance) are also freely used because of their association with "religious entities" – institutional or not. In many cases, these titles may be used by anyone with or without specific training or skills. The determination of what someone actually does when they call themselves an "energy healer" or "manifestation coach" or "light worker" or "success trainer" is elusive. All of these, including yoga teacher, may exist under the umbrella of "spiritual entrepreneur" – an individual who claims that they are engaging in a selfless vocation. Though they may have completed certifications and degrees, and even offer their own trainings, these certifications are, by their own admission, not recognised by external governing bodies, and there is little, if any, oversight to their practices or claims of efficacy. Some spiritual entrepreneurs go so far as to certify themselves through degree programs of their own making.

Doctoral degrees may be used as marketing tools because they confer prestige and are rarely questioned.[7] As Ben Goldacre describes in "When in Doubt, Call Yourself a Doctor" – an analysis of cult "group-think" and healing:

> Authority is so important with health information . . . and [medical experts] are so immaculate, so ruthlessly pedantic . . . [their] [a]uthority is a shortcut to reliable information. You take stuff on faith because reading, critiquing and checking that academic references are valid and represent the material they refer to, and more, is very time consuming.
>
> (Goldacre 2006)

It is possible for individuals to title themselves "ministers of holistic healing" conferred through their own doctoral degree programs. The association of spiritual entrepreneurship with 'ministry' is an interesting one, and it is quite common. This is perhaps, because ministries (religious orders and institutions) enjoy preferential treatment and less oversight than other institutions in American culture. As educational institutions that cannot be accredited, to confer degrees and avoid legal jeopardy, students must be ordained as ministers. Dr. Paul Leon Masters, founder of the International Metaphysical Ministry and the affiliated Sedona University and University of Metaphysics, speaks about the structure of the online universities to prospective applicants:

> Your own legal right to teach, counsel, or heal in the contemporary field of Metaphysics today is determined by having an ordained ministerial status, not upon a doctoral degree in Metaphysics. *The primary purpose of the doctoral degree is to establish a highly professional image* [authors' emphasis] of you as a person who is truly educated in Transpersonal, Transcendent, Theocentric, Holistic, New Thought Metaphysics and has taken the time to obtain a doctoral level of knowledge.
>
> For the reasons stated, therefore, you must have a ministerial status to practice legally. As explained in our catalogue, you may obtain such ministerial status through our degree program. The subjects covered in the curriculum of this course are listed further on in this catalogue.
>
> Ministerial status with the International Metaphysical Ministry is, therefore, a prerequisite for studying and earning a Bachelor's, Master's, or Doctoral degree from our universities.
>
> (Masters, University of Sedona Website)

Dr. Masters himself is said to have cautioned clients to be wary of the many "charlatans, scoundrels, and manipulators who are ever ready and eager to mislead the earnest seeker of Truth. Students of metaphysics as well as laymen should understand the difference between true spiritual metaphysicians and scoundrels assuming the title" (Paranormal Wiki 2010). Masters goes on to describe the signs of a fraud:

> One of the most apparent signs that may indicate falseness on the part of pseudo-psychics is their use of fancy titles that is supposed to reveal their "spiritual" standing. All sorts of high-sounding titles are used to impress the public concerning their so-called spiritual status or the many "powers" that they are supposed to possess. Sometimes these titles are legitimate but most often they are self-given or "purchased".
>
> (Paranormal Wiki 2010)

In sum, in the world of spiritual entrepreneurs, one must be wary of titles and degrees since training is generally unregulated, unaccredited, and aimed at those who may be vulnerable and suffering (seeking healing when Western medicine has failed them), or who are genuinely sincere in their spiritual seeking. The lack of oversight and regulation of holistic modalities requires that the consumer do due diligence to ensure that they are being trained or treated by a skilled and qualified practitioner. Organisations like Yoga Alliance are voluntary industry registries that act to promote practitioners, engage clients, and assist in the selling of services. They have no authority to police or regulate those who choose not to become members. There is nothing preventing anyone – qualified or not – from granting doctoral degrees in yoga. In all likelihood, it would prove popular since it would appear to legitimise an otherwise elusive field in the public's mind.

## MONEY FOR NOTHING, RESPECT FOR FREE

Holistic vocations may be appealing because they require little investment[8] – no formal education, few resources and, because they are so popular, there are many examples to imitate. The alleged righteous nature of these vocations is also alluring because it speaks of the practitioners' character and their desire to sacrifice for others. This sacrifice also acts as a justification should criticism be levelled at the efficacy of their practices, their work ethic, or their lack of financial success. The fierce competition for those that "need help" leads to marketing strategies that frame everyone as "ill" or "suffering". Absent needy or vulnerable individuals, these practitioners are out of business. 'Healing confessional'[9] is commonly used as a way to drum up business as it admits to the potential clientele that the practitioners themselves are grateful consumers of the same products.

Though their stated role is to serve others, there are some spiritual entrepreneurs who also enjoy financial success. Their justification for making money is well summarised in the following bit of advice offered by Susan Guillory:

> For a long time, I equated being spiritual with being broke. I'd known too many yoga teachers who struggled to pay the bills. I only saw people who weren't great at business and who prioritized their spiritual interests . . . Then during Covid, I began to meet really successful female entrepreneurs who were also spiritual. The two were not mutually exclusive. I began to understand that one could be openly spiritual *and* make great money . . . But for many people, there is often a block to overcome. Many operate from a scarcity mindset, which means they don't believe they can make a lot of money . . . and so they don't. Thoughts create reality, so for those who limit the possibility of abundance, this becomes their reality. It can take a bit of work to overcome this obstacle, but it's completely doable. And then the sky's the limit in terms of what a spiritual entrepreneur can earn!.
>
> (All Business Website)

## THE FOOT SOLDIERS OF RECTITUDE

Much of the wellness industry has come to occupy an uncomfortable territory between a pyramid scheme and multi-level marketing. According to prosecutor Letitia James, "A legitimate multi-level marketing company emphasizes reliable products or services. A pyramid scheme uses products or services to disguise its quest for collecting money from the investors on the bottom levels to pay other investors further up the pyramid" (James 2022). Unlike multi-level marketing, a pyramid scheme is a business that relies on the ongoing recruitment of new members, rather than on the products being offered. The most common way to accomplish this in yoga, and many other holistic practices, is to get clients into teacher trainings and certifications as soon as possible – often without regard for level of knowledge or skilfulness. Those at the top of the pyramid in wellness businesses need more than clients; they need to train others to carry out their mission – to convert potential clients into community members. This is endemic to the whole of the wellness industry; click on a holistic training ad on Facebook to receive a barrage of advertisements for certifications – sound healer, energy worker, spiritual coach. The successful marketing of a myriad of trainings is so abundant that practitioners increasingly have a multitude of undecipherable letters after their names. A justification for this recruitment is the notion that everyone is "spiritual" – everyone has untapped intuition and power through which they can transform the world into a more loving and enlightened place. These trainees aid in the 'groupthink' that is the ethos of their studio or practice. It is these foot soldiers that may believe whole-heartedly in the rhetoric – that they are sincerely changing the world for the better and have evolved by moving up through the levels that their practice defines. This is why the wellness industry depends so heavily on trainings. In the yoga industry, this has resulted in a glut of teachers, most of whom are enthusiastic about their brand, yet inadequately trained. After their connection to the brand, their enthusiasm is their most significant asset; they have little to teach but their "love" of yoga. This impacts on their ability to attract students which may ultimately result in disillusionment and cause them to leave the practice altogether. Training new foot soldiers, therefore, is a priority for the wellness pyramid. Foot soldiers are expected to recruit and eventually train others in an effort to expand the brand's reach and the pyramid's base. Popular strategies to recruit potential trainees are donation-based (pay what you can) or free classes/products (e.g., "just pay for shipping" or "first month of classes are free" or "91% off!") or making the entirety of the training "online" or "at one's own pace" for convenience. Novice teachers or teachers in training are commonly expected to teach without compensation to prove their dedication to the brand and to hone their skills. This may expose the weaknesses in their teaching. Typically, additional and ongoing trainings will be recommended and can add up to a significant investment (financially, time expended, emotionally). As a result of this investment, and the public nature of their proselytising, trainees and community members may be less apt to leave or question the brand, even when doubts arise. The brand and membership in the community have become a significant part of their identity. The commitment to the community builds and maintains the number of members needed to keep the brand popular, rather than the quality or efficacy of the practice or product.

Flaws found in the brand are rationalised with the justification that the practice or product is seen as working for the greater good. Despite any critiques they confront, foot soldiers take comfort in this belief. When disillusionment occurs, foot soldiers may feel betrayed and compelled to publicly announce their departure and the ways that they have been injured. This may only serve to consolidate the community because it feels attacked. If foot soldiers leave *en masse*, this may cause a crisis for the pyramid as its base becomes unstable. The brand may have to take action to reclaim its reputation by admitting to the lesser critiques and attesting to its dedication to reform. It is likely that those at the top of the pyramid are aware of what they are doing. To manage the inequality inherent in the pyramid structure, they may periodically highlight their own flaws and struggles so that they appear as equals to those below them. This also serves to reinforce the need for continuous training and the reaffirmation of the ethos of the brand. The admission of fallibility also acts as an excuse for any perceived wrongdoing at present or in the future.

Before the founding of Yoga Alliance and the flowering of the certification process in yoga and the wellness industry in general, teaching was commonly done by experienced and skilful practitioners. Though Yoga Alliance has attempted to raise the quality of teaching in the industry through its regulation of schools, these attempts are viewed by many as unsuccessful. This is especially true of individuals who were teachers before the organisation existed. The Yoga Alliance are viewed as such because adherence is voluntary, there is little oversight or enforcement of regulations, and the minimal standards that are set fall well below what was expected of a teacher in the past. It is also difficult for excellent teachers and practitioners to remain in the industry because the ease of certification has led to an abundance of certification programmes which have produced a glut of insufficiently trained teachers, many with little experience in practice. This largely results from encouragement of certification in the industry and a studio model that necessitates trainings to ensure financial solvency.

Confusion also exists between types of trainings and certifications. In the yoga industry, it is common to offer 'intensive trainings.' These are generally short, condensed sessions, where one is immersed in the subject matter. Intensives may last anywhere from a weekend to a month in duration. By contrast, one may train *extensively* with one teacher or school over the course of many years or for the duration of one's career. The ambiguity inherent in the term 'intensive', when not contrasted with 'extensive', may leave people believing that those who have taken an intensive are highly trained. However, intensives are generally meant to peak one's interest through an immersive experience – a spur to deep on-going study. When someone says they have studied intensively with a teacher and have received a certification, they could be speaking about a day-long workshop or a four-week course.

Credentialing, when it is over-emphasised and is not dependent on a formally evaluated skill set, is likely to lead to a diminished quality of training and less-skilled practitioners. In fairness, part of the overemphasis comes from practitioners themselves who seek to accumulate titles rather than, or in addition to, increasing their knowledge and skill set. A typical FAQ on online training sites is "Does this program come with credentials I can put after my name?" Professional standards mean nothing if they are not clearly understood, effectively taught, and evaluated practically. As previously stated, the business model for studios is also a problem because it relies on trainings which offer credentialing as a way to remain financially solvent. There is value in continuing to train and enhance one's yoga skillset and breadth of knowledge. It is a problem, however, when one's motivation to accrue credentials is more important than acquiring skills and knowledge. Given the above and the enormous variety of treatments or nominally therapeutic procedures that can be sold as yogic or as adjunct skills, the proliferation of certifying programmes will only continue to expand. Studios typically find that when competing in the bloated certification marketplace, over time, there are diminishing returns. Sadly, if this trend continues, the over-credentialled and under-experienced will be the norm of the yoga industry and studios will continue to struggle to stay open.

## IMPLICATIONS: THE FUTURE IS NOW

The healing power of yoga has ancient precedent. In medieval times, *haṭha* yogis used postural practice, dietary restrictions, and cleansing rituals to ward off illness and cure disease. This was accomplished under the mentorship of a *guru* and through dedicated practice. Today, yoga therapists have their own certification programs (IAYT)[10] that are meant to support professionalism in the yoga therapy industry and promote yoga therapy as a respected form of complementary medicine. In 2016, the Yoga Alliance created a policy that restricted the designation "yoga therapist" on its members' websites and listings for fear of litigation. This action was prompted by the recognition that some of its members were practicing out of scope and misrepresenting their training and capabilities. The Yoga Alliance acknowledged that teachers were using their 200-hour certifications to offer a variety of "healing services" without proper training and against ethical standards. In 2021, Yoga Alliance amended its policy to focus instead on meeting ethical and scope of practice standards (common to all professions). This has led to a compartmentalisation in yoga that now distinguishes between *haṭha* yoga teachers and yoga therapists.

"Yoga Alliance acknowledges and embraces the therapeutic benefits inherent to the practice of yoga and supports members who hold any credential that advances their growth on the path to professionalization" (Yoga Alliance Website, 2021). But is yoga an inherently therapeutic practice? If so, how do Yoga Alliance and others support this claim? If not, what factors do lead to therapeutic or beneficial results? In addition to the positive effects of the placebo response already mentioned, yoga has been marketed quite successfully as a healing modality. When polled, the general public (98%) overwhelmingly agree that yoga is good for you and that they practice or intend to try yoga because of its positive physical or psychological benefits (Saper, Goldstein, and Khalsa 2013). This is believed despite the fact that, though a significant amount of research is being undertaken, the results of this research are, as yet, inconclusive. As Saper, Goldstein, and Khalsa conclude in their study of yoga practitioners:

> Future studies of yoga may consider measuring and/or setting realistic expectations concerning the benefits of a yoga practice over the short and

> long term. There are many physical and psychological reasons why individuals begin or return to yoga, of which preventing or treating illness and achieving or maintaining sound physical and emotional health was dominant . . . While there is a growing literature on the health effects of yoga in a clinical setting, there is insufficient research at the community level among non-clinical populations, particularly data on how yoga is incorporated into daily life.
> (Saper, Goldstein, and Khalsa 2013)

Saper, Goldstein and Khalsa highlight the difference between the realities of practice in an experimental setting versus in a more naturalistic one. They recognise that yoga is a very varied practice and that *how* something is practised is as important as *what* is practised when determining its therapeutic qualities. If there are aspects of yoga that do scientifically show significant therapeutic benefits, the causal factors should be isolated to ensure that yoga is the cause of these benefits rather than simply correlated with the feeling of well-being.[11]

'Life coaches', 'influencers', and 'thought leaders' are not the same as teachers. A teacher gives instructional information about the underlying principals and applications in a discipline based on their own ongoing research and practice. The others advise clients on ways to improve their lives, give encouragement, and offer strategies for advancement. The coach is a self-employed entrepreneur who develops a career around improving people's lives. The teacher's motivation, on the other hand, is to evolve or experiment within their discipline in order to transmit this information and interest to their students. A teacher is selling intellectual curiosity, and a coach is selling the idea that one needs coaching to be "their best self" and "live their best life". The acknowledgement of this distinction between teacher and coach is vital to the future development of the discipline of yoga. Evolution requires the acknowledgement, encouragement, and admiration of teachers who are best positioned to facilitate this advancement.

Spiritual entrepreneurs refer to themselves as individuals who are motivated to help people, and this takes precedence over making money. They may also see themselves as conduits of "God's love and compassion" and say they are "creators of a better world absent the residue of trauma and fear". They advise and coach their clientele about how to manifest their "best and fullest lives" through intuitive powers, dedication to goodness, and faith. In the case of yoga, regardless of these stated aims, those who describe themselves as spiritual entrepreneurs might be accused of giving the entrepreneurship (creating a lucrative business and renown) precedence over the yoga. They often aim to expand their entrepreneurial reach by branching off into adjacent enterprises that they claim also bring spiritual advantages (e.g., energy work, essential oils, past life regression, crystals, "magick", and CBD products). The spiritual entrepreneur believes that their brand of capitalism is righteous, rather than exploitative or manipulative. They may despise capitalism while freely participating in the yoga industry. They appear to believe that what they are selling is virtuous and so it strips their financial activities of any pejorative association. They may disparage science and Western medicine but seek the kind of academic degrees associated with these disciplines.

In a time when degree inflation has become problematic, it is no wonder that spiritual entrepreneurs and others in the wellness industry seek to earn "doctoral" degrees in addition to certification. But what value do these certifications or degrees really hold? In yoga, the quality of certification and continuing education programmes varies widely. Some traditions have rigorous and lengthy training that requires passing multiple examinations offered through their governing body (e.g., Iyengar Yoga System), while others offer online or very brief trainings where everyone is awarded certification. In the future, yoga professionals may decide to go the way of others in the wellness industry and become "doctors" in addition to collecting a cornucopia of certifications. In the end, certifications and degrees do not matter in any discipline. What matters is the quality of the training one gets, the genuine dedication one has to their understanding of practice, and the sincerity with which the practitioner approaches continued exploration. What is needed is practitioners dedicated to serious study and the desire and ability to pass on what they know to the next generation of yogis.

## NOTES

1. A spiritual entrepreneur may be defined as "[to] have a knowing inside of yourself that you are here for a reason and that it is time to express the voice of your soul through business . . . [and the] desire to be of service in the world through a business that you create. – Devi Adea https://spiritualentrepreneur.com/ or "someone who runs a business in a spiritual or wellness industry . . . These entrepreneurs center their work around helping people. It's not as much about the bottom line (though they can be financially successful, which we'll talk about shortly) as it is about making an impact in the world". https://www.allbusiness.com/are-you-a-spiritual-entrepreneur-211766-1.html.
2. The belief in their special status and the rejection of the scientific method and evidence-based research is, in part, why many in the spiritual and wellness communities rely instead on their intuition and insight. The popularity of anti-vax (and the distrust of Western medicine) and conspiracy theories like *QAnon* in these communities are examples of the power of strongly held beliefs over evidence.
3. The 'sick role' in sociology was first described by Parson's in *The Social System* (1951). For a dispassionate discussion and analysis of the "sick role" see anthropologist Robert Murphy (1987).

4. Liminality is a state of transition, a threshold, between one stage and the next, especially between major stages in one's life or during a rite of passage (ritual). The concept of liminality was first developed, and is used most often in the science of anthropology, to explain the powerful ways in which rituals and ritual contexts can transform individuals and groups.
5. Those in licensed professions, like Western medicine, are also vulnerable to dependence on certainty which may lead to misinterpretations and the holding on to false theories and beliefs.
6. The term "doctor" is not even a protected term in some countries, including the United States (Goldacre 2006).
7. If a consumer does not think a doctorate degree matters, then they should question why the practitioner claims to have one at all.
8. The University of Metaphysics offers bachelor's degrees for about $250 and Doctoral degrees for $450. Each takes only six months to complete online. There are no stated prerequisites except the requirement to be ordained as a minister.
9. Healing confessionals are a part of what has come to be known as "trauma bonding" or "victim Olympics". Spiritual entrepreneurs and their clients share personal stories of trauma and the struggles that allowed them to overcome what appeared to be insurmountable obstacles. In this way, the community becomes deeply dependent on one another because they know each other's secrets perhaps more intimately than family and friends.
10. International Association of Yoga Therapists.
11. Correlation and causation are not the same thing, even though they can sometimes exist at the same time. Correlation is a relationship between two variables where a change in one variable is likely to accompany a change in the other (it is a covariance), but causation is when one thing is actually the cause of another.

## REFERENCES

*All Business*. "Are You a Spiritual Entrepreneur?" Accessed 28 August 2022. https://www.allbusiness.com/are-you-a-spiritual-entrepreneur-211766-1.html.

Brown, J. 2014. "Yoga and the Placebo Effect". Accessed 30 August 2022. https://www.jbrownyoga.com/blog/2014/3/yoga-and-the-placebo-effect#:~:text=When%20applied%20appropriately%2C%20yoga%20is,more%20than%20can%20be%20stifled.

*Delray Center for Healing*. Accessed 12 August 2022. https://www.delraycenter.com/services/yoga/.

Goldacre, Ben. 2006. "When in Doubt, Call Yourself a Doctor". *The Guardian* Fri 21 Apr 2006. Accessed 30 August 2022. https://www.theguardian.com/science/2006/apr/22/badscience.uknews.

Harvard Medical School Blog. 2022. "The Real Power of Placebos: Are 'Fake' Treatments Real Treatments?" Matthew Solan. https://www.health.harvard.edu/staying-healthy/the-real-power-of-placebos. 1 December 2022.

James, Letitia. "Consumer Fraud and Pyramid Schemes". Office of the New York State Attorney General. Accessed 29 August 2022. https://ag.ny.gov/consumer-frauds/pyramid-schemes.

Masters, Paul Leon. *University of Sedona.* Accessed 12 January 2024. https://universityofsedona.com/accreditation/.

Murphy, Robert F. 1987. *The Body Silent.* New York: Henry Holt & Co.

*Paranormal Wiki.* 2010. Accessed 12 January 2024. https//:paranormalwiki.blogspot.com/2010/04/frauds-in-metaphysical-field-part-1.html.

Parsons, Talcott. 1951. *The Social System.* Glencoe, IL: The Free Press.

Pearson, Joel. 2024. *The Intuition Toolkit: The New Science of Knowing What Without Knowing Why.* NSW: Simon & Schuster.

Saper Robert B., Richard Goldstein, SB Khalsa, and Mary T. Quilty. 2013. "Yoga in the Real World: Perceptions, Motivators, Barriers, and Patterns of Use". *Global Advances in Integrative Health and Medicine* 2 (1):44–49. doi: 10.7453/gahmj.2013.2.1.008.

Sexton, Shannon. 2014. "Healing Heartbreak: A Yoga Practice to Get Through Grief". *Yoga Journal.* Accessed 12 July 2022. https://www.yogajournal.com/poses/healing-heartbreak-yoga-practice-get-grief/.

Smith, J. Andy, Tammy Greer, Timothy Sheets, and Sheree Watson. 2011. "Is There More to Yoga Than Exercise?". *Alternative Therapies in Health and Medicine* 17 (3): 22–29. Accessed 30 August 2022. https://www.proquest.com/openview/d0e95f9d67d88557c61e355e9f965b7b/1?pq-origsite=gscholar&cbl=32528.

Swart, Robert. 2021. "Trina Campbell Wants to Bring Healing to Bodies in Detroit Through Yoga and Reflexology". 11 August 2021. Accessed 23 August 2022. https://umbrellalocalheroes.com/trina-campbell-wants-to-bring-healing-to-bodies-in-detroit-through-yoga-and-reflexology/.

*The Power of the Placebo Effect.* 13 December 2021. Accessed 30 August 2022. https://www.health.harvard.edu/mental-health/the-power-of-the-placebo-effect.

van Gennep, Arnold 1909/1977. *Les rites de passage* (in French). Paris: Émile Nourry 1909. *The Rites of Passage* (in English). Translated by Monika B. Vizedom and Gabrielle L. Caffee London: Routledge and Kegan Paul, 1977.

*Yoga Alliance Website.* 2021. "Joint Statement from the Yoga Alliance and International Association of Yoga Therapists". Accessed 13 January 2024. https://www.yogaalliance.org/About_Yoga/Article_Archive/Joint_Statement_from_Yoga_Alliance_and_the_International_Association_of_Yoga_Therapists_IAYT.

*Yoga Glo.* 11 August 2014. Accessed 12 July 2022. https://blog.glo.com/2014/08/yoga-for-healing-2/.

Chapter 6

# Why Languages Matters

Suzie Batiz of the popular wellness website Thrive Global states, "If you knew that the words you spoke became your world, you'd choose them much more carefully" (Batiz 2020).

## LANGUAGE AND CULTURE

It was once a popular notion that language shapes reality. As Benjamin Lee Whorf, famously stated, "Language is not simply a reporting device for experience but a defining framework for it" (Whorf and Carrol 1956, 212). Language, in this simplistic perspective, is a filter for reality – it shapes the way we think and determines what we think about. Whorf focused on the importance of words to argue his position, claiming that language determined culture by patterning our thoughts – the absence of a term in a language's vocabulary would, therefore, preclude the possibility of that thing coming into existence in a culture. It claims, for example, that if there is no word for "green", the experience of the colour green does not exist. But is this the case? Or is it more likely that the word "green" exists within a language because within *the culture* it is necessary to distinguish green from other colours – our culture, shapes our language and, therefore, our consciousness, not the other way around. Consider for example, the claims that in Inuit language there are many terms for "snow". This might mean that the many terms for snow allow the Inuit to perceive snow with greater clarity and, as a result, these distinctions become important within the culture. Conversely, it could support the conclusion that distinctions in snow are so important in Inuit culture that they have

DOI: 10.4324/9781003471752-9

coined a vocabulary capable of communicating essential information about their environment. From this perspective, culture conditions our thoughts and observations that, in turn, create language – the expression of these thoughts.

Other researchers have noted that linguistic structures other than words are responsible for conditioning thought. Lera Boroditsky's experiments indicate that grammatical structures of any given language can alter our perceptions (Boroditsky 2011). For example, Italians might experience the past with more exactitude because they have many more past tense formations indicating distinctions in the character and quality of what has gone before. Or the French may see the world through a more gendered lens than the English because nouns are always attributed gender in French – a system absent from English grammar.

The way that languages organise and categorise aspects of a culture's reality may *influence* the way that reality is interpreted, but it does not create it. Humans use language to create and express some sense of order in their world – they create categories which simplify reality. One often groups together words that represent concepts by their physical proximity or their similarity to one another. For example, a tomato may be a fruit or a vegetable; a blossom may be a flower or simply a weed. Things may be classified as food in one culture and not in another – dandelion, horse meat, rodents, insects, and beef – are these edible? In addition, the way we use language, and its specific meaning, is bounded within communities, most particularly in communities of practice.[1]

How then might we describe the way that language effects reality? Most linguists and anthropologists today believe that language and culture are part of a larger coevolving cognitive system. Scholars reject the deterministic and reductionist assertion that language *creates* our perceptions, culture, and reality. Language changes according to the changing worldview of the culture. Just as language cannot create physical reality, it also cannot merely reflect physical reality. It always imposes a doubly subjective vision; a vision consisting of the meaning encoded (by culture) in the language being spoken and the view of the speaker who chooses the words being used.

Language is symbolic and words are imperfect attempts to capture the complexity of the things they signify. They create cognitive categories and structure relationships among things through a process of simplification.[2] Some aspects of reality are highlighted, and others are ignored as these relationships are created. As Whorf observed, these categories and their structure then influence how we interpret sensory input (Whorf and Carroll 1956). When one comes a across a plant with a blossom they have never seen before, they will interpret it as a flower based on established categories and their important features. Yet if asked to be more specific, one can certainly observe the uniqueness and complexity of each bloom. Linguistic categories do not control our ability to perceive, but they do influence what and how we perceive in everyday experience. Language allows us to draw conclusions easily, but lacks the subtlety found in experience. This is why one often finds they "don't have words for things". Language is, therefore, an imperfect representation of reality which relies on symbols and interpretation to communicate meaning.

## LANGUAGE AND IDENTITY

Language always has social meaning. It is used to signal identity by those who speak it, and speakers are also categorised by others according to the way they use language. People belong to many social groups and have multiple social identities that they may signal through language. According to anthropological linguist Daniel Everett, language can be considered a cultural tool to relate a community's values and ideals and is shaped and moulded by people in that community over time (Everett 2012). Each group will have a 'jargon' or specific way of speaking. Intonation, verbal contour, and other paralinguistic features reflect and reinforce both cultural beliefs and identity for members of a social group. When this community is defined by a shared interest which is enacted, it is known as a 'community of practice'. In a community of practice, people learn skills and ways of thinking from other members rather than from some organising or codifying institution. One thing that is shared within a community of practice is a specific language and way of speaking. The greater the shared beliefs within a community (and therefore shared language conventions), the greater the clarity and power language can wield.

## THE LANGUAGE CONUNDRUM

In "Yoga and Wisdom: Reflections on the Body at the Intersection of Epistemology and Ontology" (2020), Joseph Alter discusses the conundrum presented in yoga where philosophical premises about the nature of reality posit an ineffable, disembodied truth which comprises "wisdom". A fundamental problem arises because *Sāṃkhyan* philosophy struggles with having to use words to describe a structure to reality that transcends language (at the level of enlightenment – pure consciousness or *puruṣa*) but nevertheless takes shape in the body of (enlightened) incarnate souls (Alter 2020, 108). Language is part of the reasoning mind (*buddhi*), which is part of the material world (*prakṛti*) – it is not the source of truth that is embodied as the "wisdom" of enlightened beings (like the *guru*). Though

*Sāṃkhya* is decidedly atheistic and logical, this truth cannot be expressed with words. As Alter states:

> . . . words are signs that signify correspondences which constitute reality by means of representation. Words are not the thing they represent; they capture it – they do not make it real as a tangible, corporeal thing unto itself. Worth their weight in gold as knowledge, words are worked by language against the very idea that truth is somehow ineffable and yet, at the same time, incarnate as wisdom.
>
> (Alter 2020, 114)

Language itself then poses a problem for yoga philosophy and the ontology it proposes. As a function of reason, representation, and the intellect, it exists outside of the truth where the wisdom gained through the experience of enlightenment resides. Wisdom, *puruṣa*, and enlightenment are "beyond words" in traditional yoga philosophy. Alter further suggests that language does not "silence claims to wisdom . . .[it] simply translates the conceit of wisdom into public knowledge within a framework of common, collective interest". Embodied wisdom, especially as manifest in the modern form of the *guru*, "is antithetical to the production of collective knowledge based on discussion, debate, disagreement, compromise, and consensus" (Alter 2020, 117). How then might we understand the role of language in contemporary yoga where we prioritise critical thinking and intellectual discernment?

## A YOGIC LEXICON

Yoga may be understood as a community of practice on many levels – studio, style, school, locality, or even worldwide. The language used in contemporary yoga (as in other milieus) is meant to reflect and reinforce shared values and beliefs of the community, in part, through specific vocabulary. Many of these terms, familiar to those who practice, are shared with the fields of cognitive and religious studies – in particular New Age religious milieus. Words are deliberately selected and used to signal identity within the community and express a set of presumptions and beliefs which underlie the terms of practice. They also serve to distinguish members of the yoga community (or orthodoxy, or studio) from those who are not. What follows is an inexhaustive attempt to identify and analyse some of the more important terminology and use of language by yoga practitioners and others in the yoga community.

### The Nature of Self

The curious use of yoga-speak to describe the indescribable is found in the discussion of the nature of self. Here, the uppercase 'Self' refers to a primal experience to be found within an individual that is seen to be identical to the primal nature of reality and a lowercase 'self' is the personal identity of an individual. The study of self and its place in reality is foremost in the minds of most yoga practitioners, whether they are in pursuit of the loftier goal of "Self-realisation" or simply looking to be "their best self" in the material world. The "foundational Self", "true Self", and the "essential Self" are common terms used to indicate the belief in some extant essence which is the primal substance of one's "true nature". This Self is believed to be present and unchanging, yet not easily accessed in the context of the material world. The "best self" is described as "balanced", "centred", "grounded", and "unchanging" to indicate its right nature. These same terms are also used to describe health and well-being – they are basic notions of natural states in both yoga and ayurveda and indicate their unwavering nature. If one grows closer to this realisation, they may speak of "growth" toward a "higher self" – one that is capable of realising their purpose in life or *dhārma*. People speak of *dharma* as an indication that they have found their purpose and understand their "calling" to be the result of their accumulated actions or *kārma*. This is believed even though *dhārma*, originally understood as one's inherent duty, is now seen as the discovery of one's singular talents and a choice to put these talents to use as a gift to others. The use of the Sanskrit terms *kārma* and *dhārma* also signals a belief in the theoretical precepts of the ancient practice of yoga. Sanskrit is believed to be the sacred language of traditional practice, and because of this, the mere use of Sanskrit terms signals membership in the community of modern yoga and knowledge of its teachings.

### The Nature of Reality

Specific words may also be used in yoga-speak to express beliefs about the nature of reality. The concept of 'energy' is central to the modern yogi's understanding of the nature of the universe, and it is accepted as the foundation of all that exists. Practitioners may view yoga as a way to access and manipulate energy for some benevolent purpose, ranging from self-improvement to "healing the world". Illness and discord may be viewed as energetic problems which require that energy be brought back into a state of "balance". Some people speak of feeling "the energy of the room" or one's "energy being off" and they may conflate these amorphous beliefs with other energetic practices. It is not uncommon to see energy balancing practices like reiki, crystal therapy, grounding, or chakra balancing integrated into yogic practices.[3] Food may also be presumed to have energy, as do thoughts and actions. Food practices, therefore, become important indicators of both one's values and one's membership within the community of yogis. Vegetarianism is so common that it is the presumed diet of yoga practitioners, and veganism (part of doctrine in modern Jivamukti Yoga) is growing in popularity. The popularity of veganism is due, in part, to the way it falls in line with yogic ideas about the singularity of sentient beings and is couched in the language of positive change. Jivamukti teachers will often end class with the chant: "We are vegans, and we are saving the world" (Gannon 2009). The same can be said of thoughts and actions – they are perceived as producing "good" or "bad" energy – the very same energy that shapes one's *kārma*. Therefore, yogis may privilege positive emotions and thoughts over those they deem detrimental, as thoughts and emotions may be manifested through energetic means.

The concept of energy is also understood in terms of the 'spirit'. Because energy is believed to exist and is viewed as a scientific fact, "consciousness", the "cosmos", "cosmic consciousness", and "universal consciousness" may be reframed as both demonstrable and measurable. The universe is understood for its energetic "expansiveness", a term referencing the science of physics. This expansiveness is also a quality found in practitioners and is seen as a measure of their spiritual awakening. To be spiritual is to be energetically expansive – to be more in tune with the universe rather than "energetically stuck". Because energy is what drives the universe, a more advanced practitioner may be able to "manifest" (make real) things energetically that they desire. The success with which they are able to manifest is evidenced by their success in their personal endeavours. With dedicated energy, the yogi believes it is possible to accomplish all that they desire in both the physical and spiritual worlds. The term energy acts as a powerful floating signifier – a term without a clear referent and no agreed upon meaning. Everything is energy. The term may, therefore, be employed and interpreted in a myriad of powerful ways to describe the nature of reality.

## The Yogic Way to Self-Realisation

There is also a lexicon that is employed to describe the yogic process for advancement or self-realisation. The self is "realised", rather than created, because (as stated above) the perfect Self already exists but has been masked by the illusion innate in the interpretation of sensory information. People speak of their practice as a "path" or "journey", indicating its importance, but also alluding to pilgrimage – an endeavour that is inherently spiritual and, in the case of "path", linked to one's *dhārma*. A yogi may be said to undertake a "sacred journey" or "true path" in seeking realisation. There are a number of ways that one might advance on this journey to enlightenment, and these are also articulated in vocabulary that has specific meaning in the context of modern yoga. Whatever the particular method, advancement in yoga is seen as an "evolution" to a more "awakened" state where one can "see" the truth. This truth is, by its very nature, masked by ignorance (*avidyā* – inability to see), both by the individual and society (who's institutions must never be fully trusted). Some yogis make a distinction between those that are on "the path" and those that instead choose to live in this state of ignorance.

One modern adaptation of a traditional path is the practice of *bhaktī* yoga in which "love" (considered a powerful embodiment of pure energy) is expressed through chanting. The equation of "love" with "god" allows secular-minded yoga practitioners to dedicate themselves to a spiritual rather than (what they view as) religious practice. The popular idea of a "heart-centred practice" is illustrative of the shift from a dedication to "god" to a dedication to "love". To be heart-centred is to be open hearted, which is undirected and associated with other yogic values like "acceptance", "compassion", "passion", "empathy", and "purpose". To be open-hearted is both energetically receptive and energetically giving, a condition ripe for "transformation". Transformation is not equivalent to change. Change looks to the past in comparison to the present, but from the yogic perspective transformation is novel and energetically created.

Likewise, the recitation of *Oṃ* is an example of the importance of energy in the process of transformation. *Oṃ* is understood as the sacred vibration of the universe, and some yogis believe that if one chants *Oṃ* perfectly, they will manifest the perfect universe, of which they are a part. Even mundane words (not in the sacred language of Sanskrit) have taken on powerful evolutionary meaning for modern yogis. Suzi Batiz explains on the wellbeing platform *Thrive Global* that "words are energy in the form of vibrations, and our vibrations create our reality", and that by "watching our exaggerations", "surrounding yourself with affirming statements", and "reframing negative thoughts to positive ones" one can "step into the role of 100% creator of your own reality" (Batiz 2020). She adds that language is so imbued with energy that:

> Over time the structure of your thalamus will also change in response to your conscious words, thoughts, and feelings, and we believe that the thalamic changes affect the way in which you perceive reality.
>
> (Batiz 2020)

Other yoga practitioners prefer more physically embodied forms of evolution. In the Iyengar system, "alignment" is said to "equal enlightenment". This assumes that if the body is perfectly aligned at the "cellular level" in postures and held there in stillness, energetic perfection is achieved, and enlightenment will spontaneously occur (Iyengar 1979).[4] Just as concepts in physics have been adopted to reframe the concept of the "universe" as science, scientific theories may be interpreted by modern yogis to legitimise the quest for self-realisation. Derived primarily from the simplification of complex theories in psychology and neurobiology, these principles, and the practices they create, aim to legitimise alchemical and otherwise unsubstantiated theories. These "scientific practices" wax and wane in popularity and are evidenced in approaches like "polyvagal therapy". Here, the vagus nerve[5], is reduced to a master switch to physical, psychological, and spiritual well-being. Lack of attention to the vagus nerve and its "tone" are seen as roadblocks to evolution, and so yoga practices aim to manipulate the vagal nerve. Similarly, "scientific" practices focus on "parasympathetic and sympathetic" nervous responses (controlling or diminishing the flight or fright response associated with the thalamus) and the "brainstem" (thought to contain all the ancient wisdom of humanity if accessed through breathing and meditation). These practices require neither a depth nor a complexity of scientific understanding.

In any case, if the path or journey is progressing, it will be evidenced by an increasing "awareness" for the yoga practitioner, an awareness that those who are "less evolved" do not enjoy. The seeker may also find increasing "abundance" that is both material and spiritual by doing "the work". Eventually, the seeker hopes to reach an enlightened state which is marked by the experience of "ecstasy" or "bliss". This ecstasy will, at first, be fleeting but will, it is believed, eventually encompass the whole of the enlightened one's being.

## Non-Judgement, Decolonisation, and Inclusion

The yoga community, wherever it exists, is a subculture of the larger culture and society in which it is contained. It is expected therefore, that many of the values, beliefs, and ideals of the larger culture will be shared in the yoga community, if viewed as promoting progress to yoga's goals. One can see the impact of cultural trends in the language of modern yoga as it reflects the concerns within the larger society. In an attempt to rationalise its practices, the yoga community has adopted the task of "decolonisation". This is in response to grander issues of equality and access, and also serves to disentangle modern yoga from claims of "cultural appropriation". A "decolonised yoga" is one that lauds Indian culture, aligns itself with the Hindu roots of practice, and de-prioritises the forces of capitalism, neoliberalism, and Westernisation. In other words, a decolonised yoga is "true and authentic yoga" (absent the atrocities wrought by colonialism). It is a way to cleanse modern Western yoga – an obvious product of colonial and imperialistic forces.

The decolonising of yoga entails that practitioners admit the errors of their past and begin to remove alien forces that have created inequality.

Yogis may now opt for trainings in "trauma-sensitive yoga", "gender-affirming yoga", and "accessible-yoga" in order to create "inclusive environments" free of judgement and the trappings of colonisation. This requires a dedication to a number of beliefs. "Non-judgement" is possibly the cornerstone of these beliefs for it asks that all things be accepted as they are – as perfect. The idea that "one is perfect the way they are" is the foundation of other moral precepts of this enlightened ideology.

## THE USE OF SANSKRIT

As has been illustrated above, the selective use of Sanskrit is fairly common in the yoga community because it signals both authenticity and authority in either practitioner or teacher. Whether denoting postures or core values and beliefs within the community, the use of Sanskrit is selective and particular. There are conventions in yoga and its various communities of practice for when and how Sanskrit is to be used. An individual practitioner's agreement with these conventions is one measure of community membership as is their ability to use Sanskrit appropriately. As few modern yogis speak Sanskrit, Sanskrit words are used independently in an act of language mixing (e.g., Sanskrit words carefully placed within English conversation) as signifiers rather than for communication. Sanskrit is also commonly the language used in chanting, and dedicated practitioners may take a Sanskrit name, or be given one by their *guru*. Sanskrit names are markers of status, again signalling authenticity. Much like Hebrew, Aramaic, Greek, or Latin, Sanskrit is found in religious contexts and is considered sacred. It is not important, for example, to understand Sanskrit when chanting for it to carry profound meaning or achieve a desired effect. The use of Sanskrit is an identity marker. It serves to distinguish yoga from other physical and meditative practices.

## KĪRTAN, CHANTING, MUSIC, AND MĀNTRA

Chanting, whether in Sanskrit or not, is often accompanied by the harmonium, sitar, drums, or singing bowls, and has become popular within the yoga community. Classes may include chanting, whether it be a traditional invocation bestowing gratitude to one's lineage found in many modern orthodoxies, or traditional chants from other devotional practices like *bhaktī*. There is also specific music for yoga, usually referring to compositions with dulcet tones and modern and ethereal voices of singers who are recognised as devotional yogis. *Kīrtan* is used to describe devotional music. This music is often upbeat and can be accompanied by free-form dancing which is also seen as devotional. It is not unlike the speaking in tongues or manifestations of "the spirit" found commonly throughout other mystical traditions. One is taken over by their spirit or their true selves during a successful *kīrtan* session. Chanting as a group may also be interpreted as a rite of incorporation, where the group affirms its common bonds and values, beliefs, and ideas – it strengthens the individual's membership in the community and the health of the community to which they belong.[6]

## Māntra

Historically, Sanskrit is viewed as a sacred language and its sounds are believed to be the vibrations that create reality. The sound, rather than the meaning of words, is of primary importance in the traditional chanting of *māntras.* Through repeated recitation and upon enlightenment, the meaning is eventually revealed – a meaning that is to be kept secret to maintain its potency. As Joseph Alter notes, "the secrecy is a process whereby insight is embodied by transforming the gross sound of words into relatively more subtle [silent] self-understanding . . ." (Alter 2020, 111–112). This is readily apparent in the value placed in concepts like *anāhata* (the unstruck sound) versus the sound *Oṃ,* that when uttered, is only an approximation of reality. As Alter states:

> The arbitrary meaninglessness of sounds in the form of mantras and dharanis is a profound reminder of the magical arbitrariness of words themselves in relation to the objects they represent. And, therefore, this meaninglessness is a reminder of the concrete reality of knowledge that is based on an understanding of how words work – semiotically – apart from the substance of things and ideas they seem to denote in a world of direct experience.
> (Alter 2020, 116)

As Alter explains, the structure of reality presented in *saṃkhyā* philosophy identifies speech as the grossest manifestation of sound. The sound of each letter in the Sanskrit alphabet is subtler than spoken words, but the meaning found at the level of *puruṣa* is where unadulterated meaning, free of the ignorance of the material world, is found. It is unspoken, yet wholly comprehended (Alter 2020, 111).

In contemporary yoga, *māntra* has been denuded of its traditional meanings and is more likely equated with a secular form of prayer. *Māntras* may be selected by one's teacher, but may be just as likely chosen by the yoga practitioner themselves. Unlike chanting or *kīrtan,* the *māntra* is seen as a deeply personal enterprise. The *māntra* is a symbol of their personal journey toward self-realisation and an indication of their progress. In a gross departure from tradition, the words of the *māntra* carry great meaning. The modern use of *māntra* may be the result of the democratisation of yoga and the loss of the sacred status of the *guru* and, in part, a measure of the greater importance placed on individuality in today's society.

## VOICE AND AFFECTATION

The "yoga voice" is an affectation that is meant to be an expression of the qualities one expects to find in a dedicated practitioner. The yoga voice is ritualised and used specifically for the purpose of teaching or talking about yoga. If teaching, it is rhythmic, keeping time with the music or pace of movement and is typically reflective of the serious and contemplative nature of practice: calm, reassuring, and with a tendency to melodrama. A common technique is to exaggerate the calling of the breath (as with "inhaaaaale" and "exhaaaaaale"). Exaggeration may also be used to inspire others to push harder, break through barriers, and "let go of their ego" or "surrender". The breathing in some styles of yoga is, like voice, an affectation, and is expected to be audible. Depending on the style of yoga and the specific breath practiced, the sound of the breath can take a variety of forms (e.g., *ujjayi*, *kapālabhātī*, or *bhrāmarī*). The audible breath has a variety of meanings. It may signal the "energetic potency" of one's breathing. In some cases, practitioners associate the volume (loudness and capacity) of one's breath to be indicative of the skill level of the practitioner and the power of their breathing. It may also be believed that less energy is expended with proper breathing, since energy is harnessed and directed to "the practice".

## NON-VERBAL COMMUNICATION AND PARALINGUISTICS

### Gesture

There are many ways that gesture is used to communicate in the yoga community. Gesture ranges from comportment of the body to the performance of various *mudrās*, each with a designated energetic purpose. When one gestures, they are trying to convey meaning with their bodies. Gesture can accompany spoken language or communicate on its own. When one feels akin to another, they tend to mimic their gestures and comportment as a natural empathic response. This results in a language of gestures specific to each community of practice.

In common parlance, *mudrās* are gestures made with the hands.[7] Although there are many *mudrās* found in tantric texts, only a few have gained popularity in modern yoga. The most ubiquitous is the "prayer position" (*añjali mudrā*), which is often accompanied by the Sanskrit utterance "*Nāmāste*" ("I bow to you") and/or a bow. It is quite productive and may also be used as a greeting, a general sign of respect, a way to open or close practice, or to be devotional (pray). *Mudrās* are also imbued with amorphous energy and alchemical properties. They are believed to change the impact of one's thoughts and actions, be it in meditation, chanting, or physical practice. Some *mudrās* are also used in *prāṇāyāma* (e.g., alternate nostril breath, and *bhastrikā*) and *pratyāhāra* (controlling the senses by closing the eyes, ears, nose, and mouth). Other *mudras* are prescribed for specific postures (e.g., reverse prayer for *Pārśvottānāsana*, or prayer for *samasthitiḥ*). *Mudras* are also thought to assist in the removal of "blockages" and restore the free-flowing movement of *prānic* energy, a requisite for health and wellbeing. Most *mudrās* are traditional, but some are of modern origin. Placing one hand on the abdomen and one on the heart (either seated or lying supine), for example, is commonly performed to connect with one's spirit.

## Body Comportment

In addition to the hands, the body is an instrument for expression. It is common for practitioners to sit or stand with a straight spine to signal their dedication to yoga practice. The straightness of the spine is associated with both physical health and spiritual attainment.[8] Other common ways the body communicates dedication are in stretching or warming up rituals which may precede a physical practice or occur at other times apart from physical work. These rituals are ubiquitous, highly personal, and usually (but not exclusively) performed on one's mat. They are performed spontaneously rather than led or prescribed.

The body is also used in specific ways for both meditation and relaxation. The most common body comportments for meditation include lotus position (*padmāsana*) and corpse pose (*śavāsana*) both executed with a straight spine. The eyes are usually closed during meditation or meditative physical practice. Functionally, closed eyes allow for fewer distractions, but as a communication, it expresses an inward turning or a spiritual striving.[9] Other variations for seated meditation are possible, but full lotus is iconic and synonymous with yoga. It is also a difficult posture, requiring substantial hip flexibility and, therefore, also functions as a powerful symbol of an "advanced practitioner". "Advanced", though ill defined, is very often used to describe a practice or a practitioner's skill in modern yoga. Typically, advanced refers to challenging postures (e.g., inversions and postures requiring exceptional flexibility, strength, or balance) and those that have the ability to execute these shapes with their bodies. It is not about experience, although advanced physical skills are often equated with spiritual attainment.

### Bodily Adornment

Dress and bodily adornment also function as forms of communication and identity marking. Some styles of practice, like kundalini, require a standard uniform, but most modern yogis carefully craft their yoga attire. Yoga pants are so popular that they have successfully exceeded the confines of the yoga studio, and modern yoga clothing is as much about fashion as function – fashion forward styles can actually impede practice. As with all fashion, different brands tell different stories about the practitioner. The more popular brands can be very costly and signal to others that one has made a serious investment in practice. Organic or ethically sourced clothing, on the other hand, signals one's moral virtue. Practicing without a shirt is acceptable for men in many yoga studios, distinguishing yoga from other fitness regimes. The amount of skin men or women expose has meaning, but one that is regulated by the conventions at each practice space. Adhering to the conventions for dress signals, once again, alignment with a specific yoga community, and practitioners can often identify like-minded practitioners by their dress.

*Mālā* beads (strings of prayer beads ended with a tassel) are common forms of adornment for yoga practitioners. Though they were traditionally used devotionally, today they may be worn as jewellery within or outside of yogic contexts. They may be wrapped around the wrist as a bracelet or worn as a necklace. The wearing of a *mālā* signals that one practices yoga. It also infers that one is spiritual. Other devotional jewellery includes charms depicting Sanskrit words, images of the Buddha or Hindu deities and other sacred symbols like the *Haṃsā*, the tree of life, or the *cakras.* Crystals are also popular adornment either worn as jewellery or placed beside one's practice space. It is believed that crystals have the power to transform energy and thus communicate one's belief in the importance of energy and one's ability to manipulate it to meet one's goals.

## THE BUSINESS OF YOGA

As a community of practice, yoga practitioners believe that their strivings are focused not only on the betterment of themselves, but on the world as a whole. This righteous endeavour risks being tarnished when yoga is viewed as a capitalistic enterprise. Practitioners in the business of yoga, be they teachers, studio owners, or therapists of some sort, therefore, may define themselves as "spiritual entrepreneurs" – those who devote their lives to the betterment of others by sharing their unique gifts. Spiritual entrepreneurs speak of ways they can help one to eliminate "roadblocks", "blockages", and energetic and spiritual "stagnation" so that one might "evolve" to be their "best self" or "highest self". They attest to the fact that each individual also has unique "gifts" that they are meant to share with others – given to them by "the universe". The neglect of these gifts (which are brought to light through their tutelage) is, therefore, a violation of universal principles. The righteous intentions of the spiritual ameliorate any stains that may result from the monetising of "the practice". This may be indicated in the language used to describe the financial exchange. It is not a fee, price, or a cost, but an "investment" or "tuition". These terms serve to help distinguish the financial exchange from materialistic pursuits and reflect the higher purpose of the service provided by the spiritual entrepreneur.[10]

## "ABUNDANCE" VERSUS "SCARCITY" MINDSET

The words "scarcity" and "abundance" are commonly used to describe one's mindset or perspective. One's mindset is important because it will determine what one will potentially "manifest" in their lives. A "scarcity" mindset stands in the way of one's advancement – it arises from the "attachments" that practitioners may have to the material world. People with a scarcity mindset can fall into a cycle of "negative thinking" focusing on what they don't have and resenting others who they believe have what they don't. Conversely, an "abundant" mindset is representative of one's achievement of a state of "contentment" – they are free from desires in the material world, allowing them to appreciate life in its fullness. As described on the spiritual site *GoodNet.org*:

> In a spiritual context, the notion of abundance or plenty is less about material conditions, revolving instead (once basic needs are met), around an appreciation of life in its fullness, joy and strength of mind, body and soul. This is the cultivation of respect for the creative energy of the universe. An abundant life is one that leaves negative feelings of lack, dissatisfaction and emptiness behind. Instead, it is open to light and love that come from a more spiritual domain.
>
> (GoodNet)

It is believed that one can shift from a scarcity to an abundance mindset and, in doing so, improve their lives and the lives of those around them. "Visualisation" is one powerful method that may be used to make this shift – visualising the life you see yourself living.

## THE YOGIC LIFESTYLE

Contemporary yoga connects practitioners through a set of shared values and beliefs. The floating signifier "yogic" can be used as a powerful reference for these values and beliefs because it evokes a number of meanings that suggest seriousness and positivity. As it lacks a singular definition, yogic is a highly useful term with broad application. Though interpretations may vary dramatically, they will still signal group membership and shared fundamental values. When one says something is yogic, they are making a reference to its positive nature – environmentalism, a focus on peace and love, a vegetarian or vegan diet (as they have respect for all living beings), and other righteous lifestyle choices.

There are other floating signifiers commonly employed in modern yoga that are highly productive in both their usage and meaning. "The work", "the process", and most notably "the practice" all assume a shared understanding of exactly what is meant in the designation "the" as well as an acknowledgement that this is privileged information. Though nouns grammatically, they all imply a timeless "doing" – they are active and eternal and, therefore, impossible to describe. "The practice" is distinguished from "my practice" and "your practice". "The practice" encompasses all that is correct in the pursuit of yogic goals although, and because, exactly what is practised lacks any specificity. One's individual practice has clarity but is trivial in comparison. Even less restrained by definition is "the work", which can be understood as the concerted and relentless effort to accomplish the difficult task of transformation. One has either "done the work", for which they are admired, or "not done the work", a sign that they have not made, and are not willing to make, the sacrifices necessary for success. "The process" describes the changes that take place during the course of yogic transformation. It can be used in the context of "the work", "the practice", or any other obstacles the yogi might face. "The process" describes what one should expect as they become more "evolved beings". It is meant to be difficult, full of trials and tribulations which test one's dedication to "the practice", and its undertaking is further evidence of the superiority of the "yogic lifestyle".

## WORDS, STORIES, AND NARRATIVES

Language in yoga makes up a larger narrative that becomes the reference for, and the context within which, personal stories and the words used to tell them are interpreted. This narrative outlines the shared values, beliefs, and assumptions held within the community. For example, a narrative may be that "when one opens their heart with compassion, then one's transformation can begin". A yoga teacher may tell a personal story about overcoming addiction through "self-acceptance" and "self-love" to support and strengthen this narrative and the students will understand the purpose of the telling. The phenomenon of such "*dhārma* talks" at the beginning of classes has become quite common in modern yoga. They serve to remind students of the community's definition of yoga and the purpose of their practice within it. Once a community has strong narratives, communication within that community is commonly interpreted through them. These narratives are not generally questioned, and their application may be outside of conscious awareness. Strong narratives allow for assumptions to be taken for granted. An outsider, or a visitor to class, may interpret the words and stories differently since they may not share, or be aware of, the community narratives.

Language is alive. It does not only exist on a page, but mainly through the interactions of interlocutors. As such, language, like the community within which it exists, is always changing. Whether through unique lexicon, ways of speaking, or gesture, the language used by the yoga community is distinctive and provides a window into the current yogic worldview. Through an analysis of the way language is used and meaning is conveyed, one can also see how effective communication is accomplished, and how the values, beliefs, and ideals of the yoga community are created, expressed, and instilled in its members. The arbitrary relationship between the vehicles for communication (words, gestures, ways of speaking) and their meaning allows language to coevolve with the changes in values and beliefs in each community of practice. Therefore, the language of yoga, at any given moment, and in any specific context, provides a way for yogic values to be reaffirmed by the community and transmitted to future generations of yoga practitioners.

## IMPLICATIONS: THE FUTURE IS NOW

Language does not create consciousness, but it may influence one's perception. What language does reveal is the values, beliefs, and identity of individuals and the communities they interact in. In particular, communities of practice share a unique vocabulary and way of speaking that is created and maintained through group interactions. Language is also a powerful shorthand for identity marking. People are rarely completely conscious of the implications of their speech. But without this awareness, there is a risk that the language of yoga may become empty and wholly performative – the metamessage ("I'm using Sanskrit to tell you I'm a yoga teacher") becomes the entirety of the meaning.

'Floating signifiers' are terms that are so potent, and so encapsulate a community's values and beliefs, that they can be used in a myriad of circumstances. As such, floating signifiers may act like 'summarising symbols' – a symbol that sums up an entire domain of meaning – or as 'elaborating symbols', which provide categories for analysing and conceptualising experience through analogy. A nation's flag is a good example of a summarising symbol because it expresses all at once everything about that nation, whereas a machine, as an elaborating symbol, may be used as a metaphor to understand the way the human body works. Floating signifiers, in yoga-speak, are much the same. The terms 'yogic', 'energy', 'the work', 'the practice', and 'the process' are all highly productive and powerful signifiers that need not be analysed for understanding to occur – though above, we present an analysis of these terms, people in the community of practice would have no need for such scrutiny. In fact, community members may struggle to define these terms precisely, even though they are well aware of what they mean.

The amorphous nature of floating signifiers makes them less subject to analysis by those who use them in the yoga community, as well as by those that don't. For example, 'freedom' could be claimed to be a floating signifier in American culture. People claim to "love freedom" or feel that their freedom is being threatened but may be hard pressed to actually define freedom or the logic of threats against it. This means that those that act in the name of freedom are never pressed to reflect on their beliefs. Is this the case for the yoga community (with terms like 'the practice', 'the work', etc.), even though the goal of the yogic lifestyle is the search for truth and self-knowledge? Because terms may go unanalysed and have broad application, there is a danger that people will fail to see the *empty* nature of these terms. It is also possible that metaphorical speech is taken literally which creates another fallacy. Concepts like 'sacred geometry', or "the body is a machine" are imaginative metaphors rather than accurate accounting of the divine nature of performing postures or the actual workings of the body. When metaphorical speech is mistaken for literal reality, it is also more likely to be left unanalysed.

Linguists agree that language is a symbolic system – the sounds of language have an arbitrary relationship to the meanings they express. Many in the yoga community share the belief however, that Sanskrit is a sacred language that lacks this symbolic nature. Each sound is said to have a unique resonance and a unique effect – its sounds *are* its meaning because reality is seen as vibrational and sounds are simply vibrations – the sound of *Oṃ*, for example, is the sound of the universe. According to the *Yoga Sūtras of Patañjali* (1:28), simply chanting *Oṃ* in meditation can lead one to a state of *īśvara praṇidhānā* (awareness of something greater than yourself or surrender to god) through a vibrational transformation – when one meditates on the chanting of *Oṃ*, the yogi becomes one with it, through the process of absorption. The belief that Sanskrit is non-symbolic is scientifically inaccurate. Sanskrit is, like any language, subject to interpretation and change, as is illustrated in its lengthy history of usage and definitional breadth. If one believes that chanting can alter the universe vibrationally then, since all languages are vibrational, it should also follow that any language could be as effective as Sanskrit.

In most cultures, sacred languages coexist in what has been termed a 'diaglossic' relationship to languages used for everyday purposes. For example, Latin (the 'high form') was used as the language of worship solely in the context of the Catholic Church, whereas Italian (the 'low form') was used everywhere else in everyday contexts. The high form is a prestige form and does not have to be comprehended by its users but affords those who use it status and power. The low form is the conversational form and its use marks low status for its users. For Sanskrit to assume this sacred nature, one must assume that it was used in a similar context of diaglossia in relation to other Indian language varieties. Houben's (2018) sociolinguistic research shows that what we consider sacred or "classical" Sanskrit was codified during the first century CE. At that time there were two forms noted in the written literature: *bhāṣya*, the "conversational form" and *Mahābhāṣya*, the high or sacred form. Preceding Sanskrit were older forms like Middle Indo Aryan. The social power and prestige of the newer classical variety of Sanskrit is apparent in the influence it has had in the development of the other languages of the Indian subcontinent. Houben calls this "linguistic paradox" a "problem" for Sanskrit scholars which has still been left relatively unaddressed (Houben 2018, 1–18). The control of a sacred language attributes power and esteem to the priestly caste and scholars that may use it. Because no one in yoga speaks Sanskrit in most contexts and it is unnecessary for the proper execution of physical practice, what has its purpose become? People will attempt to control knowledge to gain or retain power, within as well as outside of the yoga community.

## NOTES

1. Communities of practice are groups of people who share a concern or a passion for something they do and learn how to do it better as they interact regularly. Communities of practice are formed by people who engage in a process of collective learning in a shared domain of human endeavour: a tribe learning to survive, a band of artists seeking new forms of expression, a group of engineers working on similar problems, a clique of pupils defining their identity in the school, a network of surgeons exploring novel techniques, a gathering of first-time managers helping each other cope. (Wenger-Trayner, Etienne and Beverly 2023).
2. A cognitive map is a type of mental representation which serves an individual to acquire, code, store, recall, and decode information about the relative

locations and attributes of phenomena in their everyday or metaphorical spatial environment (Tolman 1948).

3. For an in-depth analysis of the conflation of energy work amongst modern practitioners see Bender (2010).
4. BKS Iyengar states "True alignment means that the inner mind reaches every cell and fiber of the body." (Iyengar 1979)
5. "The vagus nerve represents the main component of the parasympathetic nervous system, which oversees a vast array of crucial bodily functions, including control of mood, immune response, digestion, and heart rate. It establishes one of the connections between the brain and the gastrointestinal tract and sends information about the state of the inner organs to the brain via afferent fibers." (Breit, Kupferberg, Rogler, and Hasler 2018).
6. For more discussion about the value of chanting and its role in group consolidation and feelings of belonging see "What Really Matters" in this volume (Chapter 4).
7. There are also *mudrās* made using the entire body (e.g. *mahā mudrā, or sarvāṅgāsana*), but most practitioners think of *mudras* as hand gestures. In either event, traditionally *mudrās* are like *bhandas*, understood as "energy locks".
8. In most traditions, the spine needs to be straight for enlightenment to occur through the ascension of *kundalinī* energy up the central energetic channel (*suṣumnā*).
9. Most traditional facial expressions are no longer commonly practised in modern yoga. (e.g. the *tantrika* gazing up cross-eyed at the "third eye" in the center of the forehead, or the accompanying protruding tongue in Lion Pose). The authors feel this is due to the fact that yoga practitioners are highly cognisant of their appearance, and find these expressions look unattractive or silly.
10. For a more detailed analysis of spiritual entrepreneurs and the wellness industry, see "When Credentialling Doesn't Matter" in this volume (Chapter 5).

## REFERENCES


Alter, Joseph. 2020. "Yoga and Wisdom: Reflections on the Body at the Intersection of Epistemology and Ontology". In *Capturing the Ineffable: An Anthropology of Wisdom,* edited by Philip Y. Kao and Joseph S. Alter, 103–121. Toronto: University of Toronto Press.

Batiz, Suzie. 2020. "Your Words Create Your Reality – So Choose Them Consciously", in *Thrive Global.* Accessed 4 January 2023. https://community.thriveglobal.com/your-words-create-your-reality-so-choose-them-consciously/.

Bender, Courtney. 2010. *The New Metaphysicals: Spirituality and the American Religious Imagination.* Chicago: University of Chicago Press.

Boroditsky, Lera. 2011. "How Language Shapes Thought". *Scientific American* 1 February 2011. Accessed 2 June 2023. https://www.scientificamerican.com/article/how-language-shapes-thought/.

Breit, Sigrid, Aleksandra Kupferberg, Gerhard Rogler, and Gregor Hasler. 2018. "Vagus Nerve as Modulator of the Brain-Gut Axis in Psychiatric and Inflammatory Disorders". *Front Psychiatry* 9: 44. Accessed 2 April 2023. https://www.ncbi.nlm.nih.gov/pmc/articles/PMC5859128.

Everett, Daniel. 2012. *Language: The Cultural Tool.* New York, NY: Pantheon Books.

Gannon, Sharon. 2009. "Satya and Veganism". *Jivamukti Yoga* February 2009. Accessed 2 June 2023. https://jivamuktiyoga.com/fotm/satya-veganism/.

*GoodNet.* 2020. "Spiritual Abundance as a Positive Response to Our Current Challenges". Accessed 3 February 2023. https://www.goodnet.org/articles/spiritual-abundance-as-positive-response-to-our-current-challenges.

Houben, Johannes. 2018. "Linguistic Paradox and Diglossia: The Emergence of Sanskrit and Sanskritic Language in Ancient India". *Open Linguistics* 4 (1): 1–18. Accessed 17 June 2024. https://www.researchgate.net/publication/325230910_Linguistic_Paradox_and_Diglossia_The_emergence_of_Sanskrit_and_Sanskritic_language_in_Ancient_India.

Iyengar, BKS. 1979. *Light on Yoga.* New York: Schocken. Revised edition.

Tolman, Edward C. 1948. "Cognitive Maps in Rats and Men". *Psychological Review* 55 (4): 189–208.

Wenger-Trayner, Etienne and Beverly Wenger-Trayner. 2015. "Introduction to Communities of Practice". Wenger-Traynor.com. Accessed 2 June 2023. https://www.wenger-trayner.com/introduction-to-communities-of-practice/.

Whorf, Benjamin Lee and John B. Carroll, eds. 1956. *Language, Thought, and Reality: Selected Writings of Benjamin Lee Whorf.* Cambridge, MA: Technology Press of Massachusetts Institute of Technology.

*Yoga Sutras of Patanjali.* 2012. Sri Swami Satchitananda. Yogaville, VA: Integral Yoga Publications. Revised edition.

SECTION III

# THE TRANSMISSION OF KNOWLEDGE

*Chapter* **7**

# The Empathic Dilemma

In yoga circles nowadays, it has become *de rigueur* to be an 'empath' – empaths are seen to be superior because of their assumed greater intuition, sensitivity, and compassion. However, people are not empaths – empathy is a state in which people operate, to varying degrees, in different circumstances. Simply put, empathy is a skill for gathering information about others that may assist in a variety of social interactions. The powerful feeling of empathy presumes a true understanding of another's emotions. It is an undeniably pro-social skill. It does, however, have its limitations – limitations that when ignored may lead to misunderstandings and false conceptions.

## EMPATHY AND LEARNING

When considering the process of learning (in yoga or elsewhere), a skilled copier is different from someone who learns empathically. Empathic learning functions through a give and take, where the student considers the teacher's presentation and mindset and then imagines themselves as a rendition of it. Through empathic awareness, one imagines themselves as living/experiencing something, rather than copying rote what they see. It is half "this is what I imagine they must be feeling", and half "this is what I would feel". In doing so, the imitation becomes more than a skilful copy; it becomes a thoughtful interpretation of another's emotional experience. It guesses at another's inner life through what is displayed outwardly – the comportment of gesture, posture, facial

DOI: 10.4324/9781003471752-11

expression, or even sound. As education researcher Terry Heick contends:

> The role of empathy in learning has to do with the flow of both information and creativity. A dialogic interaction with the world around us requires us to understand ourselves by understanding the needs and conditions of those around us. It also requires extended critical thinking and encourages us to take collective measurements rather than those singular, forcing us into an intellectual interdependence that catalyzes other subtle but powerful tools of learning.
>
> (Heick 2022)

Self-discovery is an important way of learning and, for empathy to work, we need the ability to feel for ourselves before we can have empathy for others. For example, when you move slowly through a *vinyāsa* sequence as a means of self-exploration, you are learning the skills that you need to observe similar feelings in others. In learning, students attempt to project a more competent version of themselves derived from the model presented by the teacher. They begin to impersonate someone who they believe has superior knowledge. In this process, they should recognise that they are using their imagination conjecturally to align their genuine emotions with that of the teacher, whose emotions they can only imagine. Teachers who recognise this attempt to present an idealised version of themselves; highlighting their personal *skills* rather than their personal *life* (the parts irrelevant to what is being taught).

## THE DYNAMICS OF EMPATHIC OBSERVATION

So, what is an example of the dynamics of empathic observation? There is a distinction between simply demonstrating a skill and inviting someone into the experience. At one level, this is about the "volume of consciousness".[1] The teacher must let the students into the performance of what is being taught; not talk at or past students or give a performance for themselves. Like writers who attempt to compel an empathic response from readers by employing a variety of literary devices, teachers may use paralinguistic features (e.g., tone, voice quality, rhythm) to promote this interaction, but it is more easily accomplished using one's whole body and physical proximity in conjunction with speech. There are people who are skilled adepts at yoga, yet who fail as teachers because they are unskilled at communicating information and there are others who excel at communicating information, even though they may fail to physically execute it. To learn from the former, a student must make a greater effort – be more imaginative and make more empathic overtures. They extrapolate from the emotionally meagre presentation (which may be rich with information) – they imagine what the teacher should be feeling and then use this projection to enact their own version of the experience.

One of the ways to enhance the teaching and learning dynamic is for the student to put themselves into the physical positioning that the teacher models – assuming the same comportment. In particular, facial gestures are indicative of emotional state and there is research to show the importance of facial gestures and their association with empathy. According to Iain McGilchrist, the ability to read and imitate facial gesture corresponds to a high degree of empathy (McGilchrist 2010, 244–249), and studies have shown that people who receive *Botox* injections and lose the ability for natural facial expression may similarly lose the ability to feel and express empathy (Cairns 2019).[2]

> In a sense, communicating with someone who's had Botox is like communicating with a static image – much of the body language involved is silenced. Considering that body language, mostly consisting of facial expressions, makes up at least half of any message being communicated, this is a significant loss . . . But this facial paralysis also inhibits the ability of the Botoxed to mimic the facial expressions of others, which is critical in the formation of empathy. Facial micro-mimicry is the major way we understand others' emotions. The more deeply one enters into empathic interactions, the more profoundly one comes to understand another's experience. Both the teacher and the student need to interact in this space and the teacher who holds themselves aloof, as a pinnacle of knowledge, no matter how brilliant, may be ineffective if they fail to make themselves available in these interactions.
>
> (Cole 2013)

As illustrated in the example above, without the concerted effort of the student, some of the knowledge of the most advanced physical scholars is difficult to access. Because the desire to understand a teacher who is aloof requires the increased use of empathy, and empathy requires work, there is more likelihood that a student will be attracted to a teacher who appears to be giving them everything in an easily digestible format. Those who lead their teaching with an invitation to empathic engagement appear more accessible and also require less work on the part of the student. This is commonly seen when teachers begin a class with a highly personal story or revelation. Such intimacy might sway the student into believing that there is a close and caring relationship between them. This may enable the teacher to manipulate the student, especially if the teacher is charismatic. A person who is charismatic attracts, inspires, or fascinates other people through various means including their ability to express empathy and expand their volume of consciousness, which draws their audience close. When taken to the extreme, as cult leaders know, it is easier for the disciple to just follow, rather than do the work of learning. *The Guardian* notes in an account of a cult murder:

> Scholars who study new religious movements tend to be sceptical of the idea that people who join such organizations are brainwashed or coerced; rather, they're spiritual seekers drawn to gurus with compelling and attractive world views – "visions of a better world or of higher states of consciousness", Susan Palmer, a researcher at McGill University, told the Guardian . . . Charismatic leaders with a knack for rhetoric "capture your imagination and take you on a journey and also make you feel that they care about you and that you're close to them", Palmer said. "I mean, I've felt it listening to leaders whom I totally disagree with – I still feel swept up in it".
>
> (The Guardian 2022)

Though the average yoga class or studio is far from a true cult in its functioning, the example serves to show the potential power of emotional interchange in the manipulation of others, and points to the complexity of empathic understanding. In the *guru/śiṣya* relationship, there is, ideally, a complete empathic interaction between the teacher and student. Students may describe the experience of being in the presence of the *guru* as a feeling rather than a meeting of rational discourse. The learning experience is both highly intimate and intense. The relationship can easily be misunderstood by either the *guru* or their disciple as being more important than the outcome of study. Their empathy may facilitate an enthusiasm for the subject but should not take priority over the endeavour.

## THE COMPLEXITY AND NUANCE OF EMPATHIC UNDERSTANDING

Empathy can also be fickle; it is not experienced or applied equally in all circumstances. It is subject, for example, to what may be called the 'the cuteness effect', where people are known to be more likely to show empathy for babies, animals, or people that are attractive. "Empathy can be easily manipulated" (Prinz 2011, 226) – people who show emotions are likely to receive more empathy from others. Likewise, "empathy can be highly selective" – it is easier to have empathy for those who seem more like us. "[E] mpathy is [also] subject to proximity effects . . . [and] to salience effects" (Prinz 2011, 227). Empathy requires that the event be relevant and be bounded in time and space. When an event lacks constraint in place or duration, one is likely to experience 'empathy fatigue'.[3] Certain emotions are also more easily caught from others. Sadness, misery, and distress are the emotions we are more likely to catch when we are concerned about another and these emotions are likely to inhibit, rather than promote, interaction (and therefore learning) (Prinz 2011, 220).

While considering the process of learning, there are three ways to think about degree of understanding. The least understanding comes when something is 'copied'. This is analogous to copying a friend's answer to a math problem. The copier knows the answer and may remember it, but not the process through which it was solved. When a yoga student copies but only observes the surface aspects of the physical material rather than internal states or processes entailed in executing it, it is absent empathy. The next level of understanding is 'imitation' where the student tries to approximate the actions or ideas of the teacher. There is an attempt to evoke the teacher's way of demonstrating the material. True 'understanding' occurs when a student analyses and then interprets the teacher's information and embodies that information in their own unique way. This involves both critical thinking and empathy which ensures that the student understands the material. Learning occurs in copying or imitating however, this is unidirectional – it comes fully formed from teacher to student. According to Terry Heick, real empathic learning entails "walking around the meaning of something" so that you can see all sides of it before the interpretation is made (Heick 2022).

## EMPATHY AND RITES OF INTENSIFICATION

In groups, empathy may act as an important amplifier of connection. Such emotional contagion is reinforced by the commitment of each individual to the collective feeling (or expression of feeling) of the group – 'group-feel'. The ritual operator controls the ritual process by manipulating actions and objects (components of the ritual) that carry special meaning. In this context, the objects and behaviours are interpreted through symbolic (rather than everyday) meaning and this meaning is emotionally charged. The fact that everyone is participating enables an individual to more easily commit to the ritual actions – the manipulation of symbols allows for groups to make meaning of their reality collectively – either reaffirming or transforming their collective beliefs, behaviours, or understanding. The ability to share empathy makes this reaffirmation of group identity or 'intensification' possible. Because of this, rituals are powerful tools for group affirmation. In teaching, emotion and repetition, enhanced through ritual action, may serve to facilitate deeper learning through collective empathy. Rituals may enhance the feeling of cohesiveness within a group and, thereby, a sense of community is formed through the completion of successful ritual action. This strong feeling of community is the result, in part, of the heightened opportunity for empathic engagement in ritual contexts. This releases some of the "burden of individuality" (Nevrin 2008, 134) and also assists in the process of learning.

## THE CONTAGIOUS NATURE OF EMPATHY

Sociologist Susan Palmer suggests that the positive response to a charismatic leader is real; so real that she is surprised to see it in herself, despite her knowledge that it is manipulative. She also sees those who follow a *guru* as "seekers" who are looking for a more utopian existence of a higher level of experience or consciousness (Palmer 2001). What may be underestimated is the need that these followers have for group membership (as opposed to the charisma and rhetorical acumen of the cult leader). A cult might be understood as a community of like-minded individuals who join an institutional structure that is much like any formal or accepted church. Palmer herself, as an ex-Mormon, expresses this attraction to group belief manifested under the control of the charismatic individual. Others may have the same yearnings but reject group membership or the standardisation of ideas. She is not an apologist for cults, but an admirer of the collective strength of an order's beliefs, rituals, doctrine, and rules that govern group behaviours. The attachment is to the group rather than the leader. The group is their reality and to leave it (although they may also fear the leader) is frightening. In such instances, the group is a more important focus than the endeavour and their collective empathy becomes a force for both feelings of belonging and compliance.

For the yoga teacher, the capacity for empathy is useful to understand the emotional state of others and their difficulties with practice. It aids the processes of effective communication. It is not however, something that should be made foremost in one's teaching since it may invite a level of intimacy or agreement that is misleading. Intimacy may occur as a natural reaction to a strong emotional state in a student, but the wise teacher evaluates the emotional response and then moves on in a way that emphasises the learning objectives. By contrast, compassion may be understood as the ability to do what is in a student's best interest despite potential emotional difficulties. For example, if a student felt compelled to do an extra *caturaṅga daṇḍāsana* every time it was conceivably possible, a compassionate teacher might pull that student aside and ask them why they felt obliged to do so.[4] Empathically, the teacher may feel the frustration of the student and fear hurting their feelings. The student, confronted with their failing (a rejection of their *caturaṅga daṇḍāsana* superiority) may feel hurt, and leave the studio or teacher altogether. This is a risk that the compassionate teacher takes because they are offering information that will help the student in the long term (e.g., to avoid shoulder injuries, or to understand that difficulty or physical strength does not equate with superiority). In other words, compassion is not always kind or easy to administer, but it is the right thing to do. In contrast, emotional states may be deliberately evoked in a student from situations potent with deeply held "feelings" (e.g., a traumatic event or a known vulnerability). If sentiments are invoked, they should be in the service of teaching. Emotional intensity does not necessarily make for salient experience.

The ability to empathise, while lauded, is not of much use except as a starting point in the process of learning – where information is gathered. For example, a common empathy exercise is to have students pair up and imitate their partner's comportment. This allows each participant to mimic the affect of their partner and gather information on how they feel in their body. Gathering information is not the same as expressing care or forming a connection; care is expressed because there is interest in another's progress. This information must then be translated into action that encourages learning. If the example given above was in a yoga teacher training, the students may take the information gleaned (physical and emotional) to assist their partner in correctly executing an *āsana*. It is of primary importance to address the task at hand rather than the emotional state of one's partner. This is because emotional states are transitory and addressing them directly may invite inappropriate intimacy, evoke an elevated emotional response, or otherwise hamper learning.

Some people are emotional and expressive, but this is not synonymous with empathy. People who show a high degree of empathy may avoid social interactions where emotion or expressiveness are demanded because they are shy, timid, or even reclusive. They may also be a person who feels strongly but who is not demonstrative. There is a difference between sensitivity and empathy. People who are sensitive are said to be able to feel more, be more caring, and more empathic as a result. Sensitivity, however, is a function of the nervous system, whereas empathy is a product or tool of social interaction. Overly sensitive people may be so enrapt with *their feelings* (physical or emotional) that they fail to notice anyone around them. Their lack of ability to control their emotions is the issue rather than their capacity for empathy.

What teachers really do when they instruct is teach students how to learn, rather than imparting information directly. Many teacher trainings fail to teach trainees how to teach students to learn. This begs the question of whether teachers in training are learning themselves, or if they are simply repeating (imitating) what they see in their teacher (to later repeat this imitation to their students). Empathy is about gathering information so that one can best engage in social interactions whether they be intimate or not. Each social interaction has a different goal. The vast majority of these interactions do not benefit from engaging emotionally unless that is the objective. In learning situations in particular, engaging with or openly recognising another's emotions may actually undermine rapport.

## IMPLICATIONS: THE FUTURE IS NOW

The empathic experience is so profoundly affecting that what is undergone is easily misattributed to yoga and, cathartic though it may be, it is merely an *assumed* shared feeling with another. One may feel sad, for instance, in a fashion that they believe is synchronous with others, but that is hardly possible. They can only feel sad in the way they themselves feel sadness. Though this may provide some self-knowledge ("How do I emotionally respond in sadness?"), it remains an effort of self-invention premised on a projection of what another feels. Mimicking the emotions of others is not an activity that has a well-defined place in yoga's essential pursuits.

While empathy may not be an exact replication of the emotion of another, it unquestionably is a creative stimulus. What it does provide is an alternate perspective on reality. By provisionally assuming the feelings of another, we see reality from a convincing point of view. The level of invention and the intensity of the emotion are powerful. It feels *authentic* – it bespeaks integrity. *This is the empathic dilemma* – powerful and authentic though the experience feels, it is an experience invented within the self which only purports to be the feeling of another. It remains a highly stimulating act of projection whose uses are found in the way it fosters assumed engagement. The invention tells more about oneself than it does about the other.

When we engage in exploration, whether it be of the self or of the Other, the drawback with the explicit is that it is already known – its representation in our mind is concrete. The implicit is what we intuit; something we create from what can be inferred – it is what we sense derived from what we know. Things we sense are implied – we see a brightly coloured yoga outfit and our attention does not stop at the clothes and marvel at how they move about. We infer that there must be a person wearing them (not a machine) and that their aesthetic predilections include a liking for colourful apparel. We see "through" the explicit garments to the implicit being wearing them. We do not appreciate this in a neutral way, instead, we also quite unassumingly incorporate our own notions about colourful clothing into our creation of this implicit being. If this person has tears welling up because they are receiving criticism from the teacher, we do not just focus on the moistening eyes, we see through the outer explicit signs of their upset and form a conjecture of their inner world. We may invent narratives of how happy that person had felt wearing their colourful outfit and the tragedy of how their day has now turned so unhappy. But the empathy we feel is broadly conjectural and is founded upon our own experiences of wardrobe choice and teacher criticism and is guided by a holistic impression of the many circumstances of this context. The dilemma is that the emotional content, because it is based upon our own experience, leads us to assume an understanding that, while highly inventive and connected to the situation, is not as accurate as we suppose.

Though empathic reading, or the expression of empathy, may have some value in the process of learning, neither have much to contribute to practicing/doing yoga where the opportunity for studying others is limited – there is little opportunity to engage in the empathic mimicry of the postural tonicity of others. The physical adjustments we make to experience what we believe others are experiencing requires us to assume the postural tonicity that we perceive in them (see "Minding the Body", this volume, Chapter 1). Empathic responses are the result of one reading the subtle language of the body of another. We bring our bodies into positions that echo what we perceive. This empathic process also helps to facilitate the facial mimicry that is used to feel and express our concurrence. The emphasis on reading facial cues is uniquely human, however, other parts of the body are equally expressive. Though most research focuses on the primacy of facial expression, more recent studies have shown that the whole of the body is expressive of emotion and that when reading the body of another, a larger portion of the brain is activated.[5]

Even though there is little opportunity for personal interaction, the empathic process is not shut down during practice. The process will likely still occur, but the reciprocity is between oneself and the rest of reality – it is akin to the melding with the Other. When doing yoga, the postural attitudes of the body are holistic expressions where each part of the body fundamentally contributes. Yoga postures fall broadly into three categories: (1) postures involving the lengthening of the front of the body and/or the lifting of the chest (e.g., backbends), (2) postures which fold in on themselves (e.g., tortoise or forward bend), and (3) postures that are balanced in their execution – not moving outward or inward (e.g., simple lotus or headstand). Generally, the outward expansiveness of the first type of postures lends itself toward affects like joy or confidence – towards things apart from oneself. They are extroverted. The second show an inward turning and inhibit displays of expressivity. They are introverted. The third are deliberately neutral – an expression of a delicate balance that neither moves in nor out – stillness. The pursuit of this third option (and to some extent the second as well) may, in the past, have led to and reinforced the idea that yoga is a solitary pursuit because it is trying to neutralise or minimise the body's engagement. Yet, when we are interpreting something as immense and ineffable as reality, we anthropomorphise it – we engage with it and attribute it evocative meaning through our postural attitude, driven by our capacity for empathy. We emotionally respond according to the version of reality we have created. Contemporary yogis, therefore, can choose to practice in a way that either utilises this natural empathic ability or attempts to subdue it.

The realisation of one's insignificance before the awesome leads one to appreciate how small we are before the vastly greater magnitude of reality. This feeling of smallness provokes empathic receptivity (reading) in practitioners rather than broadcasting (expression). Yet, the recognition that one does have agency is important. We do not just interpret and express the emotional states of others – as soon as we sense the emotional state of another, we generate and broadcast our own emotional information. We can be the originators and generators of experience too. Merleau-Ponty says we do not see paintings as much as see *according* to them (Merleau-Ponty 1964). The empathic process we experience between people is also what we experience in aesthetic appreciation. Though we may be deceived if we believe our emotions are the same as the person we empathise with, we are certainly trying to see, or feel, according to the way we believe they are feeling reality. If we just see items as things, we objectify them and do not attempt to mingle our understanding with them. The *knowledge* of an object – the dry categoric facts about it – is different from an *understanding* that we have when we identify with it. This is potentially one great aim of yoga – to view the rest of reality as something with which one experiences the accord of understanding.

## NOTES

1. The 'volume of consciousness' is a description of the extent to which we extend our awareness into space. The volume of consciousness may be directed to one individual, or expanded to fill the space one occupies.
2. fMRI studies by Hennenlotter and colleagues: "demonstrate that facial feedback modulates neural activity within central circuitries of emotion during intentional imitation of facial expressions. Given that people tend to mimic the emotional expressions of others, this could provide a potential physiological basis for the social transfer of emotion"

   Subsequently, Havas and colleagues found that injection of botulinum toxin into the forehead slowed reading speed and inhibited the emotional responses of subjects to emotional passages of text. This is thought to be because engaging with the emotional component of text requires activation of the mechanisms (muscles of facial expression) for experiencing the emotions, supporting the views of Charles Darwin and William James in the 19th century.

   Further research by Neal and Chartrand has confirmed that botulinum toxin blocks the perception of, and empathy for, the emotions expressed in the facial expressions of others (Cairns 2019).
3. People are more likely to recognise and reach out to help in situations that are close to home or familiar. Similarly, they may initially show empathy for a crisis situation, but tire of this "caring" if the crisis is ongoing or appears without resolution. This is the case whether the crisis is a personal conflict (friends' relationship troubles) or on a global scale (an ongoing military conflict).
4. The same can be said for any behavior by a student that does not conform to technique and will impede their progress or cause injury, e.g., kicking up into

inversions, falling into flexibility rather than working with resistance as in lunges, splits, or backbends.

5. Citing research, B. de Gelder notes that " . . . viewing whole-body expressions elicited a wider network of brain areas compared with faces, including other areas previously associated with perception of facial expressions, such as STS . . . When affective information is conveyed by bodies and faces, overall there is comparably more activation for bodily expressions than for facial expressions" (de Gelder 2009).

## REFERENCES

Cairns, Will. 2019. "Botulinum Toxin: The Paralysis of Empathy". *Insight* 38. Accessed 14 September 2022. https://insightplus.mja.com.au/2019/38/botulinum-toxin-the-paralysis-of-empathy/.

Cole, Jessica. 2013. "Botox Silences Women's Faces – and Freezes out Empathy in Body Language". *The Guardian* (22 May 2013). Accessed 14 September 2022. https://www.theguardian.com/commentisfree/2013/may/22/botox-silences-womens-faces-empathy.

de Gelder, Beatrice. 2009. "Why Bodies? Twelve Reasons for Including Bodily Expressions in Affective Neuroscience". *Philosophical Transactions of the Royal Society London B: Biological Sciences* 364 (1535): 3475–3484.

Heick, Terry. 2022. "Empathy is an Elevated Form of Understanding". *TeachThought.* Accessed 11 September 2022. https://www.teachthought.com/learning/role-of-empathy-in-learning/.

McGilchrist, Iain. 2010. *The Master and His Emissary: The Divided Brain and the Making of the Western World.* New Haven: Yale University Press.

Merleau-Ponty, Maurice. 1964. "Eye and Mind". In *The Primacy of Perception,* edited by James E. Edie, 159–190. Evanston, IL: Northwestern University Press.

Nevrin, Klas. 2008. "Empowerment and Using the Body in Modern Postural Yoga". In *Yoga in the Modern World,* edited by Mark Singleton and Jean Byrne, 113–139. New York and London: Routledge.

Palmer, Susan. 2001. *Caught Up in The Cult Wars: Confessions of a New Religious Movements Researcher.* Toronto: University of Toronto Press and Long Reads. Accessed 15 September 2022. https://longreads.com/2013/09/28/caught-up-in-the-cult-wars-confessions-of-a-new/.

Prinz, Jesse J. 2011. "Is Empathy Necessary For Morality?" In *Empathy: Philosophical and Psychological Perspectives,* edited by Amy Coplan and Peter Goldie, 211–229. Oxford: Oxford University Press.

*The Guardian.* 2022. "Two Women Allegedly Lured a Driver to Death. They May be Part of a Fringe Sect". In US news, *The Guardian.* Accessed 11 September 2022. https://www.theguardian.com/us-news/2022/sep/11/alabama-women-lured-driver-death-university-of-cosmic-intelligence.

Chapter 8

# Myths and the Negotiation of Reality

## MYTHS AND METAPHORS

Myths are sacred or secular tales that explain big questions about the world and the human experience within it. They manipulate time and space – the necessary foundation for human experience – in uncommon ways and, therefore, signal they are meant to be interpreted poetically. As poetry, myths have the potential for broad application and interpretation. This is distinct from the vernacular usage of myth defined as a falsehood that is proposed to be true. Legend and myth are often conflated or poorly distinguished. Here, legend is defined as grand stories about supposed historical figures that share a moral, philosophic, or ethical dimension often based on mythic ideas. Narratives are stories that present a series of related events or experiences. Institutions and individuals create narratives about themselves which aim to influence the way that they are perceived and promote a particular point of view or set of values. Such narratives may be based on mythic ideas, on historical events, or wholly fictional accounts, but unlike the themes of myths, these stories are premised on the knowable. Narratives may evolve into myths or legends when time allows them to be accepted as part of tradition (in a community or culture), but this would entail replacing their "factual" components with poetic ones. Some might argue that Christ and Mohammed were important historical figures who took on mythic proportion, for example. The same might be said for Patanjali, the author of the *Yoga Sūtras of Pantañjali*, who is mythologised as a serpent with 108 heads.

Foundational myths, present in all cultures, are called origin myths. Origin myths answer fundamental questions about the nature and origins

DOI: 10.4324/9781003471752-12

of the universe and underlie a culture's worldview – their perspective on reality. Myths serve to explain universal questions about human origins and also their shared mortality. When people die, they seem to disappear and mythic attempts to account for this suggest "they go to the land of the ancestors", or "heaven" or "hell" or are "reborn" according to cultural conventions. In addition, myths explain or justify the realities of everyday life – things like inequality, values and beliefs, and natural phenomena. They authenticate the claims and actions by cultural and spiritual leaders and are invoked by political institutions to justify their strictures. A myth needs a story to serve these important functions, yet mythic stories are double edged. They elucidate if understood as symbolic tales that define and affirm the values, beliefs, and ideals of a culture or community and they produce metaphors through which we better understand the complexities of our world. However, if treated as literal truth, myths do not allow for alternate ideas; they resist change and limit creative exploration.

Metaphors may be understood as symbolic associations that lack obvious referents; they are used to make sense of things that are not readily understood or quantifiable. Metaphors are employed in myths to give meaning or clarity to the elusive nature of the unknown. Because the poetry of the words and ideas offer a range of interpretive meaning, metaphor and myth help to offer clarity in the analysis of the unknown.

Myths have figured prominently in the evolution of yoga throughout its uncertain history. The myth of Śiva and his many incarnations and roles is an example of the malleability of myths and the ability of their metaphors to explain seemingly incongruent realities. Indian lore contends that Śiva began as an outcast (*vrātyas*) having become fully enlightened and retreating from the world to the forest. Later Brahmanical interpretations speak of Viṣṇu's concern that Śiva should instead fulfil his *dhārma* and so is given a wife (Pārvatī) to bring him back to the life of a householder. Once his familial duties are completed, he may then resume his ascetic pursuits. When married, Śiva is said to have taught the postures of yoga to Pārvatī so as to join them in cosmic union; and later to a group of *rishis* who brought the knowledge of yoga to the rest of mankind. This story serves to reconcile tensions between the *Śaiva* renunciates (those that violate caste rules, the "dog eaters") and the *Vaiśnava Brahmins*; for adherence to caste rules and regulations ensured the proper working of the cosmos. This Brahmanical interpretation of Śiva as the *ādiyoga* (original teacher of yoga) serves to justify the ascendance of classical yoga and the philosopher yogis while still maintaining social and political power. In this same way, modern myths and their metaphors attempt to explain ancient lore by translating and reinterpreting seemingly conflicting worldviews and fantastical events. Modern yoga *gurus* and scholars use mythical narrative to support contemporary social and political beliefs much like the

*Brahmins* did. The potency of these myths and metaphors determines how effectively they integrate yoga as a valued endeavour and develop the practice of yoga in modern society.

A fundamental yogic belief is the possibility of, and striving for, immortality. The origins of this belief, and the mythic stories of hermit yogis that have lived for centuries without food or water, are not surprising, for the question of post-death experience is a subject of all human cultures. The idea that death can be overcome is the rationale for some of the more outré yoga procedures. The body must be overcome first by overwhelming its infirmities and then by "dying" – at least, figuratively – to be "reborn" into knowledge of the eternal and indestructible. Yet, prior to this destruction of the body, there are efforts made to achieve an adamantine hardness (Satchitananda 2012, 3.46), an elimination of disease (Vasu 1996, 4.18), and a destruction of all sorrows and sins (Vasu 1996, 4.48). With this understanding of the immortal, comes a comprehension of natural phenomena so that one can perform supernatural feats (*siddhis*). The ability to walk through objects, know everything at once, understand all languages, and have the strength of an elephant are all claimed to arise as the adept becomes immersed in practice.[1] These claims lack believability in the modern world, so this myth has been altered to fit contemporary worldviews and sensibilities. Today, one might speak of special powers acquired in yoga, like improved health, or increased youthfulness, intuition, or empathy – concepts that do not test believability for modern practitioners (but which may be equally unattainable). Analysis of developments in yoga's mythic evolution is useful for understanding historical continuity, but if one views myths as fixed and unchanging, they fail to account for yoga's continued evolution.

## YOGA REFORMATION AND REVITALISATION

When Luther sought to revivify the church, he addressed the idea that authenticity did not lie in merely following prescribed forms of religious ritual. Rather, these rites were meant to be at one with the inner world of devotion. Clearly, the worship of statues or wooden crosses would not satisfy this unless it was understood that there was a metaphoric resonance felt – that the divine was somehow present in the mnemonic device of the statue or cross. Yoga philosophy and practice share a similar conundrum – the inner life of the devotee (their subjective disposition) must be correct (directed toward spiritual discovery) for the physical practice to be more than mere physical exercise. Otherwise, postural practice simply becomes a sensual delusion (since the senses can only deliver an imperfect version of reality)[2] doomed to fail in the effort to coalesce with the inner realm. Likewise, if yoga is to be a living practice, its procedures, symbols, and precepts must speak to realities of contemporary practitioners and not ossify or memorialise the prescribed forms of the past.

Within the anthropological scholarship on culture and religion, there is a common phenomenon known as 'revitalisation'. Revitalisation movements occur when a culture or community loses their power or feels threatened by compelling forces of change. In an attempt to save their worldview, purge themselves of foreign (or other unwanted) influences, and re-establish their authority, these cultures and communities harken back to a halcyon time (real or imagined) when things were uncorrupted. These 'nativistic revitalisation movements' resist the forces of change and the ideas whose rising popularity threaten their own. Fundamentalist movements are prime examples of this phenomenon. Religious fundamentalist doctrine highlights the corruption brought on by modernity (be it Western or otherwise) and aims to eliminate what are perceived as alien ideas and lifeways. Fundamentalist doctrine commonly subscribes to literal and immutable interpretations of foundational texts. These texts become the script through which they justify their conservatism and supress alternative interpretations. The categoric dimension of authenticity in yoga is seen as embracing the "truth" of historicity and a recognition that there is "falsehood" in the yoga that has evolved in the 20th and 21st centuries. Today, there are some yoga fundamentalists whose reaction to the corruption of yoga is a nativistic revitalisation. They aim to affirm the validity of ancient knowledge, and the fall from grace that has followed, through reference to myths like that of the *Kali Yuga*.[3] Since Vivekananda presented at the Chicago Parliament of Religions in 1893, this fall from grace has been associated with the physical practice of yoga and the Western influences beginning with British colonialism.[4] The respect for academic rigour, and the lack of alternative explanations, leads yoga teachers, Hindu religious practitioners, and others who have a vested interest in yoga and its practice, to endorse these same mythic beliefs as incontestable truth.

## THE POTENCY OF IMAGERY

One example of fundamentalist thinking is the insistence that Sanskrit is vibrationally sacred and likened to the "word of god" – a literal vibration so subtle that without accurate pronunciation its meaning will be lost or sullied. The utterance (sound) of Sanskrit *is* the meaning – the arbitrary (symbolic) relationship between sound and meaning, found in *all* other spoken languages, is claimed to be absent. This fundamentalism is expressed within certain lineages who will not allow newcomers to chant for fear they will pronounce the Sanskrit incorrectly (and face unforeseeable consequences). But all scholars agree that language is fundamentally symbolic. Regardless of any onomatopoeia, words have an arbitrary relationship to their meaning, a meaning that inevitably shifts over time, especially if the language is still spoken.[5] In addition, words may have competing, or even contradictory meanings (and pronunciations), which is also the case with Sanskrit. Consider the meaning of 'yoga' – it has been variously defined by Sanskrit scholars as "union", "connection", "addition", "accession", "total", and "junction" (Online Sanskrit Dictionary 2022). Even within the canon of yogic texts, yoga has competing definitions – "the stilling of the movements of the mind" (Satchitananda 2012, 1.2), "skill in action" (Johnson 1994, 250), "a technique which stops death" (Sinh 1996, 2.16), "the practice of non-attachment" (Johnson 1994, 6.15), or "evenness of mind" (Johnson 1994, 2.48). In essence, there is no justification for understanding Sanskrit as different from any other spoken or written form of language or communication. To suggest otherwise is today indefensible. Yet, amongst yoga fundamentalists, it remains an essential precept – Sanskrit is sacred and its meaning, like its pronounced sound, is unchanging and its interpretation unquestioned.

Another difficulty that yoga's fundamentalists or literalists face is the apparent implausibility of a central yoga myth – that there is a never-changing realm (*puruṣa*) beyond the material world (*prakriti*), and one has no way to experience it with the mind or the body. It can be likened to an experience of the divine (something not of this world) that might happen only once one has abandoned (through practice techniques or divine grace) their sense of individuated selfhood. The metaphorical understanding of the structure of the universe articulates a philosophy of the nature of reality – that all that is matter; the material world in which we participate – is unable to ever perceive an alternate realm of reality that is "pure consciousness". The techniques that will take an aspirant toward this realm, however, are said to deliver extraordinary physical consequences (that must not distract the aspirant) such as miraculous overcoming of disease, age, and the limits of physics and the natural world.[6] Yet, the potency of this myth is undermined by how far it deviates from what we know about physics – just as the miracles of various religions become similarly suspect. One has to believe the impossible or one must accept that it is meant to be taken poetically – it is meant as an imaginative metaphor. Myths are meant to explain through the apparent verisimilitude of their analogy, however eccentric it may seem.

Sāṃkhya philosophy for the nature of reality is mythic in stature. In an effort to reduce reality to a singularity that accounts for everything, it is however, almost barren of imagery. This dearth of imagery remains influential in many of the ways yoga is practised to this day. For example, one of the arguments for styles of meditation that look inward, using *pratyāhara* techniques to limit the sensual imagery the body provides, is that it is seeking a foundational Self that is not sensually created or influenced. Sāṃkhya avers that if one can successfully parse away the accretions and misconceptions of reality that the senses provide – 'involution' – one will arrive at something foundational and unchanging. This foundation is supposed to be the same for everything in existence.

Yoga may be ready to concede that the nature of the universe is, instead, perpetual change as our modern understanding of physics suggests. If that were so, it could be expected that the nature of new myths and metaphors would account for this. However, as in Sāṃkhya philosophy, in contemporary yoga, Self is still believed to have some kind of foundational state that does not change. Expressions like "best self" as in "be your best self" or a "true self" or an "essential self" all have association with the mythic "Self" of *puruṣa* – an undying, eternal, and indestructible pure consciousness – something that is metaphorically evocative, but difficult to experience. This myth has also been reimagined to better align with Western individualism. The foundational Self (*puruṣa*) from which everything arises is now imagined as the individual or ego self – a self that has traditionally been understood as illusory. This individual self is believed to be immutable, discoverable, and subject to ongoing refinement – and the trappings of all one is *not,* are now seen as the source of illusion. Self-realisation (a merging with the source) is today understood as the ability to realise one's self absent the veil of societal judgement, expectations, and other impediments to personal freedom and happiness.

Even though Sāṃkhya theory of the nature of reality is difficult to defend or test, if explored imaginatively, one can step away from fundamentalist interpretations. In the same way, a dancer, through the imaginative application of their technical skill, portrays an animal such as a lion for the sake of narrative, not so that they are believed to be a real lion. Instead, they abstract elements of movement (a sinuous strut) and psychological elements (courage) that they synthesise into a complete whole so that their behaviour in the choreography illuminates a particular meaning or perspective. The nature of contemporary yoga practice does little to facilitate the chameleon-like performative or transformative skills that a dancer or actor needs – skills that may require one to move in ways that are *not* like oneself. Yoga today examines self-potential – an idealised version of what you already are – not how your imaginative capabilities elucidate the Self. It has few tools to challenge fundamentalist thinking.

## THE SOLAE

One of the curiosities of discourse on modern yoga is its general reliance on Patañjali's *Yoga Sūtras* as the "classical" text. The actual date of writing (or compiling) is notoriously difficult to pin down, but the earliest put forth suggests 4th century BCE. Even this early date is certainly well after the time of the Buddha and Mahavira (24th Tirthankara of Jainism) who both evidently studied yoga, and the populations of the Harappan civilisation who are speculated to have done so. Yoga had a long history of practice (and, presumably, philosophy) that the *Yoga Sūtras* bring together in a diverse compendium. The *Yoga Sūtras* are composed of 195 aphorisms (short strings of words used as a shorthand – often in odd order without conjunctions, derivation, inflection, or determiners). The terse nature of the verses leaves much open to interpretation by each *guru* or scholar for their disciples. And interpret they do since the average translation of the *Yoga Sūtras* is largely explication. It is possible that there are also later interpolations to the accepted text (SN Dasgupta posits the whole fourth chapter is a much later addition, [Sinha 1990, 56]), so the suggestion that it be taken as an Ur-text of yoga that can be followed and which represents a whole and perfected practice and philosophy is suspect. Its completeness and comprehensibility may not be important for, undoubtedly, the *Yoga Sūtras* are found inspiring by many because of this same flexibility of interpretation and the lack of alternate texts that promote coherent overviews of yoga. Only the *Bhagavad Gītā*, through rewriting or restatement, might represent a challenge, though it has not been incorporated as much into modern, popular yoga writing. But if either of these texts are to be held up as standards by which the yoga practitioner of today measure their own level of authenticity, they really are facing the kind of challenge that Luther faced in his attempt to revitalise religion (and hopefully they will avoid the peculiar excesses that his followers wrought in the Reformation).

Luther articulated three keys (*solae*) to belief that explain authenticity in worship, and these may also be relevant ideas for an entirely atheistic yoga. *Solae scriptura, solae fides*, and *solae gratia* refer to scripture, faith, and grace. As far as scripture goes, it is perfectly acceptable for yogis to invent interpretations of the *Yoga Sūtras*, but this should only be done when guided by experience. The physical experience of the *siddhis*, for example, "Practicing samyāma on the pit of the throat, there is a cessation of hunger and thirst" (Satchitananda 2012, 3.29) should not occur because the text avers it, but rather because it arises naturally in practice. Reality is the experience itself. It becomes authentic because of deep engagement with this process, not because of the literal propositions in the *Yoga Sūtras*. The interpretation of "By self-control over the maintenance of breath, one may radiate light" (Satchitananda 2012, 3.39), for example, can provide motivation for advancement in practice, but its power lies in its imaginative process and faith in the possibility of extraordinary experience.

The chanting of *māntra* or the recitation of Sanskrit can be equated to Luther's view of ritual recitation of prayer in Latin – understanding does not matter so long as it is heartfelt. The doctrine implied by the text recited however, must make sense. Modern practitioners may find themselves compelled to accept the doctrine of the *Yoga Sūtras* simply because of its reputation and the lack of alternatives in yoga scholarship. Without heartfelt faith or deep scriptural understanding, a practice becomes barren, lacking the grace of spiritual interaction. Luther suggested that extraordinary spiritual experience was possible, but it did not come from rote following of the rituals. The scriptures had to have a valid doctrine so that the faith was not misapplied. The problem with the *Yoga Sūtras* is that, while it proposes imagistically extraordinary things, as plausible doctrine, it fails at the level of common sense and application. No one, for example, has achieved any of the *siddhis* suggested in chapter 3, except on the level of imagination or metaphor.

*Adiaphora* is a Lutheran concept that maintains that it does not matter what a practice consists of, as long as it satisfies the three *solae.* The thing that makes yoga authentic is similar – it is deeply embodied, it is imagistically pure, and it brings about an experience of grace. This is why it doesn't matter what posture or system one practices. One can put any affect into it that they want. What matters is the rigor of the doctrine and the strength of its symbols and metaphors to invoke whole-hearted commitment to one's practice.

## THE TYRANNY OF THE WORD

There is a certain distrust of the physical practice because of the transience (and ultimate decay) of the body – whereas "the word" does not change or become corrupt except in interpretation. But where exactly are the activities referred to in texts like the *Yoga Sūtras* to take place if not in the body? What rules (e.g., lack of movement) are enforced to ensure that the word rules? Without a grounding in the embodiment of the lived world, the words or suppositions created around a text like the *Yoga Sūtras,* become diminished to a self-referential whirl of ideas. Similar to yoga, the post-modern art world could be said to be less about the art and more about the catalogue. The art, being unable to speak clearly, requires definition through what is written about it rather than the visceral affects it achieves without conceptual explanation. But obviously, challenging contemporary art can be experienced prior to the interpretation found in the catalogue. First and foremost, yoga is meant to have an effect; it is meant to be felt. There may be explanations or conjectures to come afterwards. Texts like the *Yoga Sūtras* may be useful for contextualising experience, but it would be misconceived for it to be used as the way to define yoga prior to it. Whatever doctrine may be derived from its words is an individual matter. A yoga fundamentalism derived from it, however, is as fallacious as the fundamentalism that comes from strict adherence to religious scripture. The power and applicability of these texts comes from their imaginative grandeur and their mythic proportions – their ability to inspire, not their exactitude.

## MODERN MYTH AND THE FUTURE OF YOGA

There are modern myths that account for the realities of contemporary yoga without rejecting its origins. One common and prolific myth is the power of yoga to heal. This myth spawns narratives that present individuals who are miraculously released from suffering, trauma, or physical decline through the dedicated practice of yoga. These stories serve to give authority to elite practitioners, teachers, and orthodoxies. BKS Iyengar claimed to have suffered from rickets as a child and, by his own telling, it took a number of years for him to heal his body through practice techniques before he could move on to higher yogic pursuits (Iyengar 2009, *Enlighten Up*). Bikram Choudhury, a former body builder and Mr. Universe, claimed to have been crippled (unable to even walk) before he met, and was cured by, his *guru* Ghosh.[7] Stories of healing after trauma, drug addiction, mental illness, and physical impairment abound in modern yoga and are generally accepted as illustrations of yoga's power to transform.

Another set of modern legends gives authority to particular orthodoxies. These harken back to origin myths to describe the discovery of the secret ancient systems, the rediscovery of "lost" knowledge, or trace a practice or *guru* through lineage back to a righteous source. BKS Iyengar is said to have descended from the lineage of the sage Ramanuja.[8] Krishnamacharya is claimed to have acquired the *Yoga Kuruṇṭa* (the ancient texts of Ashtanga Yoga later taught by K. Pattabhi Jois) during a pilgrimage to the Himalayas and the solitary cave dwelling yogis who resided there in a state of *samādhi.* This text, written on banana leaves, was said to have documented the ancient system, but later was eaten by ants in the cellar of the Mysore Palace (Singleton 2010, 8, 184–186). These legends serve to perpetuate the conservatism of yoga practice, since they support orthodox practices and institutions, but also because they are predicated on the myth of the singular "truth" of ancient wisdom and the necessity for a documented connection to that lineage.

Pilgrimage itself is mythic – the leaving behind that which is safe to journey to a sacred locale. The more modern take employs "journey" rather than pilgrimage and is played out in various narrations. For some, this sacred journey is about returning to Mother India; for others it is an explanation for the trials and tribulations one encounters in life. In either case, the journey is difficult, but ultimately beneficial, as the knowledge acquired through struggle is transformative. On such a journey, one traditionally encounters celestial or supernatural beings who hand down sacred knowledge. Today, practitioners look to mere mortals – their teachers and celebrity yogis – and the curated experiences they provide (e.g., retreats, workshops, and teacher trainings) for significant knowledge. These teachers are often seen as the upholders of true knowledge (like Viṣṇu for Brahmins) and/or as renegade outsiders (as was the case for the mythic Śiva).

As previously mentioned, yoga is said to result in special powers for those with a dedicated practice. The development of empathy and intuition are claimed to be signs of these special abilities. These abilities are seen as an indication of self-improvement and have become the reinterpretation of Self-realisation – which is now self-realisation – the ability to be one's best embodied individual self. This self-realisation, in the lived earthen body, is accomplished, in part, through a related belief in the powers of manifestation. This suggests that if one devotes their thoughts with sufficient intention to something, they will actualise it – whether it be wealth, that dream job, or world peace. The idea that one can influence something so all-encompassing is accomplished, in part, by a shift to a scientific worldview, where a sentient supernatural entity (God) has been replaced by a sentient scientific entity (The Universe) of equal ethereality and omniscience. Unlike a supreme deity, who is implacable, potentially punitive, and impossible for mere mortals to manipulate, the benevolent universe responds to the heartfelt desires of those who are both part of it and implore it. This is also buttressed by the preference for philosophies of personal agency popular in individualistic Western worldviews, in contrast to the more fatalistic beliefs found in Eastern cultures. In Eastern traditions, humans are believed to be at the mercy of ancestors, caste, and even a myriad of animitistic or animistic supernatural entities. In the West, one's fate is not determined, but thought to be in reach. At the same time, because humanity is part of the universe, the universe is viewed as benevolent – it "only gives you what you need". The re-interpretation and re-creation of myths and their metaphors are made to reconcile ancient or accepted beliefs with one's modern worldview and reality. The myths that evolve to move yoga and its techniques into the future will either need to reconcile or reject the contradictions that arise when one tries to accept different beliefs and behaviours that conflict with their own lived experience.

## FUTURE MYTHS

The evolution of yoga myths and metaphors will result in the rejection of some cherished legends, narratives, and beliefs. A myth is "generally regarded by the community in which it is told as both sacred and true. Consequently, myths tend to be core narratives in larger ideological systems" (Oring 1986). When beliefs are viewed as antiquated, new explanations are created to reconcile or reject them. For example, as yoga is today understood as a *spiritual* rather than *religious* practice, myths about the deeds of celestial beings have lost their mythic status. Stories about Hanumān or Gaṇeśa have become folklore – they are more akin to fables or moral tales than myths. The scientifically demonstrable Universe has replaced the indemonstrable concept of deity, just as toxicity and trauma have superseded ignorance or sin. Modern theories about suffering have yet to fully evolve mythic status. Existential fear about the repercussions of violence against nature and the narrative about its impact on the environment is presently coalescing. Traditional and modern ideas may be reconciled through reason (altered to agree with modern cultural beliefs) despite apparent conflicts.

## Illumination, Corruption, and Connection

Illumination, the fallen or corrupt, and the Self which is not distinguished by duality are themes that figure prominently in yoga mythology, and which also remain present in the yoga culture of today. The fascination with enlightenment (understood through the metaphor of illumination) is found in everything from the titles of texts (*pradīpikā*[9] is translated as "light" or "lantern") to imagining the body as a radiance of energy. Joseph Campbell, the great 20th century populariser of myths, remarks that "[t]he Indian yogi, striving for release, identifies himself with the Light and never returns" (Campbell 1991, xv). Modern works, such as BKS Iyengar's *Light on Yoga* (1979) or Dona Holleman's *Dancing the Body of Light* (1999) convey the contemporary notion of dispelling the darkness of ignorance through the *guru* (remover of darkness) by shining a light upon the subject. Light (and darkness) are symbolically potent in the culture of yoga today. Light is equated with knowledge and goodness, whereas its foil, darkness, represents ignorance and evil. Today, yogis ritualistically practice in a darkened space. This phenomenon may be an attempt to find an inner light or inner truth, through the diminishment of external stimuli. This mythic theme may be expressed as "you are surrounded by ignorance (darkness) and this malevolent reality may only be conquered through the harnessing of one's own illuminating resources" (authors' own thoughts). Even though darkness must be overcome, it is used as an aid to evolution, since it masks distractions which may waylay one from their pursuits. Darkness may also be seen as a symbolic womb in whose safety one is free from scrutiny and may be reborn. Darkness is needed to find the light. The ambiguity of darkness as a metaphor adds to the liminality of the ritual and makes the potential myth particularly potent.

The idea that our age is a fallen one – the *Kali Yuga*; an age of darkness and discord – is concomitant with the striving for illumination. One aspect of this fall is the assertion that spirit has been tainted by materialism. The scourge of materiality may, however, be ameliorated through yoga and other righteous endeavours. Though one may buy and wear expensive yoga gear, or charge high fees for classes and workshops, they need not necessarily be sullied by consumerism or commercialism, for they perform in the service of others. The rallying cry of the contemporary spiritual entrepreneur is "Don't be afraid to make money by serving people!" The possession of expensive clothing or jewellery is justified through the practice of 'nonattachment' – a modern interpretation of a foundational doctrine in the *Bhagavad Gītā*. If you have no attachment to things or actions, there are no ill effects. However, materialism and the luxuries of consumerism are also defended as ways of asserting "self-love"; a critical aspect of "self-care", especially if the purchases are righteously produced. Organic, fairtrade, and cruelty-free products are not simply free of the attachments of commercialism, they also serve to help those that are in need.

Another mythic theme is that universal toxicity is a result of the fallen nature of humanity and is a product of modernity. Toxins exist in everything – the food we eat, the images we view, the relationships we have, and even the thoughts we think. The potential for the body to accumulate toxins (*āma*) and the necessity to remove them through burning or cleansing techniques (relying on a well-tuned *agni*) lies at the heart of Ayurvedic medicine. The removal of toxins is also an ancient rationale for a physical yoga practice. The techniques for physical practice (including *āsana, śāṭ kārman, prānāyāma,* and *māntra*) remove toxins (through the removal of blockages – psychological, physical, or energetic – *granthis* – and through the stoking of ritual heat – *tāpas*) and facilitate a healthy life. Ancient yogis (naked and covered with ashes) made pilgrimages to the snowy Himalayas and defied the impact of the extreme temperatures through the internal production of *tāpas.* Modern beliefs have transformed *ritual* heat into *actual* heat, as is evidenced in the preference for heated environments for practice. It is believed that this heat assists in the transformational process through the release of toxins in sweat, even though, traditionally, sweating was antithetical to practice, for it was felt to drain vital energies.[10] This modern belief persists even though sweating depletes one of minerals (not toxins); rather, the liver is the filter for toxins in the bloodstream. These examples illustrate the power of toxicity as a metaphor for what ails society today, and the belief that actual heat (not symbolic heat) is what burns it away and leads to healing.

Modern yoga has also embraced the ancient philosophy that "all is one" – an expression that once referred to the belief in the nonduality of the Self. Today, the subtle concept of a Self that is the same as *Brahman* (*Ātman* = *Brahman*) – where there is no I or the Other, has found expression in the near ubiquitous idea of community. The central importance of community is reinforced through metaphors of belonging. Sociologist Emile Durkheim described a modern social structure as functioning through 'organic solidarity' – differentiated parts united through social exchange and material interdependence. In Western culture, individuality is prized, and this creates inherent conflict amongst individuals as well as between individuals and the society. Societies create 'integrating mechanisms' (e.g., institutions like churches, schools, political systems, and common interest organisations) to address these conflicts and promote group solidarity and integration. The more diverse and complex the society, the less perfect this integration is, and belonging becomes a critical issue for its members – described by Durkheim as a state of "anomie" (Durkheim 1964). Combatting this disconnection and sense of loneliness becomes a powerful motivator of behaviour, and it is no wonder that studios successfully market "community" to their "tribe", more readily than the actual yoga practice. The metaphor of tribe explains the degree of intimacy and connection that is expected of its members and also indicates their shared worldview. The community at the studio acts as an integrating mechanism (a machine metaphor) where unique individuals can unite for a singular purpose.

### Trauma, Surrender, and the Power of Numbers

Another myth that has been retained in modern yoga, albeit in an altered form, is that past trauma is the source of much of our present suffering. This belief about trauma is substantiated by the popular conceptions of the workings of *kārma* – the myth that past experiences and actions pattern who we are, and that what we are is fixed until this trauma can somehow be released or liberated (as from the wheel of *kārma* or *saṃsāra*[11]). In the contemporary version, trauma is not resolved through nonattachment (the *Bhagavad Gita*'s solution to *kārma*), but through a surrender to it. It is only through the acceptance of the damaged self that liberation from suffering (healing) might begin. Practices like Yoga Nidrā, Restorative Yoga, and Yin Yoga[12] have evolved to accommodate this desire for surrender. In Yin Yoga for example, practitioners passively hold deeply executed postures for long periods of time, potentially causing great discomfort. One object of the practice is to remain still in the face of discomfort and adversity and give in to the forces which are beyond one's control. Through this surrender, trauma is revealed and released, but never completely, for trauma is also a badge of honour, a sign that one has overcome obstacles, a war wound, a scar that always remains. 'Trauma bonding', where practitioners share their stories of past and ongoing suffering, has become a regular practice in both studios and teacher trainings. Whereas traditionally an Iyengar Yoga class would begin with the sharing of injuries with the instructor (so they might address these in practice), classes may now begin with the teacher sharing their story of personal trauma, or the trauma of another, as a moral tale. Iyengar Yoga uses their troubles talk to bolster its reputation as a form of medicine. Medical history is needed so that the teacher might address each student's needs with a particular "prescription".[13] Trauma bonding uses troubles talk to create relationships within the community, aver common heroism in the face of trauma, and to identify the need for release. The sharing of trauma is appropriate because it is believed that everyone has experienced trauma (life is suffering is a central metaphor in Buddhism) and remnants of this trauma will linger even after one practices techniques for release. Like toxicity, trauma becomes a simple explanation for one's suffering; as with all univariate theories (that look to a singular cause for complex phenomena), the myth of trauma is elegant and seductive and makes sense within the larger cultural narrative. Trauma could also be interpreted as the modern version of original sin. We are born into a shared inevitable suffering, and we must devote ourselves to this suffering and to its continuous and never-ending resolution. In part, the metaphor of suffering is potent because the suffering is ours; a response to the foreign invader – toxicity. To be toxic is a sign of one's personal failing; to be traumatised is evidence of one's perseverance in the face of insurmountable suffering.

Another mythic belief, popular in modern yoga, is that resistance is the enemy of fundamental change. It suggests that because the world is beyond one's control, the way forward is not to overcome or avoid obstacles, but to surrender to them. Resistance, it is believed, results in anxiety. The theme of surrender is foundational in Abrahamic traditions where the supernatural is all knowing and all powerful, making resistance to the unfolding of events futile. The futility of resistance is also found in Buddhist traditions popular within the yoga community. In Vipaśyanā meditation, "pain x resistance = suffering" – therefore, if one removes resistance, they may have pain, but without suffering. This stoicism in Eastern practices is based on the underlying metaphor that life is suffering. In the West, it is more likely that the notion of surrender arises from feelings of helplessness in the face of uncontrollable and unfathomable global forces. In this context, surrendering becomes a technique to ease one's anxiety by removing the need for agency. It also fits well with the notion, popular in traditional yogic tropes, that stresses the necessity for the dissolution of the ego. It is this same ego that resists forces larger than oneself.

Scientific knowledge is heavily predicated on numbers. In modern Western cultures, quantifiable data is generally perceived as unassailable ("statistics do not lie") and so may take on mythic significance. Numbers may be used as a convenient way of saying "this is unknowable" (e.g., the purported combinations possible in a Rubik's Cube).[14] At other times, numbers present the opposite – a boundary up to which we can set the range for knowability (e.g., beginning of the universe – how close in time can we estimate what was occurring immediately after the Big Bang). These concepts are difficult to practically imagine, so they are represented as numbers – but although they have accuracy of a kind, they are imagistically impoverished. Imagining our consciousness (or our bodies) fitting into a Planck length of time, or a commensurately small space, might be an amusing and creative exercise (see, for example, the movie *Tron*) but of questionable accuracy. Concepts like $\pi$ or $\infty$ confound the claims that numbers are precise symbolic accounting of quantities or values. They exist conceptually and are powerful in their applications but are not fully quantifiable. Quantification of the unknowable, no matter what the purpose, is metaphorical and so, the mythic power of numbers remains. Because yoga has adopted the idea that health can be measured and evaluated numerically, quantification as a measure of health and well-being is taking on greater significance. Yoga therapy research measures things like the reduced cortisol levels that attest to states of relaxation, reduced blood pressure, and increased lung capacity. Health was previously based on how one felt – it was evaluated as a phenomenological experience. Now, health is accurately evaluated in quantified measurements that may belie how one feels. In an attempt to understand consciousness, modern practitioners are likely to turn to quantifiable measures of brain activity (EEG) rather than ethereal descriptions of an undifferentiated Self (*puruṣa*). The self (the unique individual) is understood as measurable and knowable through technology even though the mechanisms of individual consciousness are seen by most to be as ineffable as the workings of the supernatural.

Both numbers and poetic imagery can be useful metaphors when imagining a version of either the individual self or pure consciousness. Because we retain mythic ideas subliminally, the metaphors associated with them propagate our understanding through analogy of all that is latent in reality. Like a seed that has the potential to germinate, blossom, fruit, and then wither, these metaphors also have latent within them a vast number of permutations. Reality – all that is other than self and that also may include Self (pure consciousness) – is an infinitely vast and permeable presence within which the self has many potential interactions. The imagery found in myths allows us to see through time so that we may not only experience the now, but also imagine what it has the potential to become. A flower perfectly embodies a flower and its resultant fruit may eventually also be apparent as a part of its nature. The myth provides a construct within which all of reality's potential is understood – it is a representation of a culture's worldview. There is nothing that happens in reality that is not interpreted through a mythic construct. Myths' endurance stem from the human need to explain the nature of reality and their place within it. This may account for why many ancient yogic myths still persist amongst contemporary practitioners, albeit with modern metaphors. The mythic construct presents practitioners with a framework to guide their interactions with reality. Through their interpretation, they play out variations on the myth (affirming their worldview). The individual, through their actions, becomes significant because through their interpretation of reality, they have a hand in creating it.

## IMPLICATIONS: THE FUTURE IS NOW

Myths are tales that explain the unknown. They provide an answer to questions that cannot be completely understood by other means – "[they] present an image of the universe that connects the transcendent to the world of everyday experience" (Campbell 2003, 7). In doing so, myths create or employ important cultural symbols and metaphors – comparisons to what is known or understood – in order to answer questions about the ephemeral.

Cevantes' famous work, *The Wit and Wisdom of Don Quixote* (Cervantes 1867) may be read as both tragedy and comedy. Quixote creates a fantastical vision (narrative) of who he wants to be. He strives to achieve this vision, but without self-knowledge, he ultimately fails – it is after all an "impossible dream". At the same time, Quixote, the visionary, is oddly worthy of respect. Don Quixote may be "crazy", but he believes in something and lives his life accordingly. He imagines possibilities that others do not. These possibilities, framed in his noble knighthood, drive his passionate quest. One might see the ancient yogis as such quixotic figures – looking to escape death by merging with an imperceivable yet ever-present consciousness. Like Quixote, the *hātha* yogis roamed from place to place, but naked and covered in ashes, a sign of their foolishness akin to Quixote's suit of armour. Just as Don Quixote saw possibilities others did not, the yogis strove to surpass the experiences found in everyday life.

Wisdom is a practical intelligence largely acquired through experience. It is the learning that results through efforts to cope with our human condition – the source of wisdom is lived experience. Our narratives should provide a vehicle for exploring the world currently beyond our reach, though how far is the quixotic question. As Cervantes warns, Don Quixote is seen as a mad idealist, but " . . . the maddest of all . . . see life as it is and not as it should be" (Cervantes 1867). Useful narratives and myths strike a balance between idealism and pragmatism. On the one hand, our stories should, like Quixote's, be visionary – they imagine places we have not yet been. Though Don Quixote may seem deluded, his fantasies allow him to follow a pilgrimage through which he eventually gains wisdom. But this is Cervantes' dilemma – at what point does idealism become insanity – get in the way of pragmatism (the ability to *reasonably* accomplish something) – and conversely when does *rationality* stand in the way of discovery? At the very least, to exceed one's expectations, one must imagine the possibilities.

The particulars of a myth are seen as belonging to individual cultures, but their universal function is to explain time and space. "In the beginning" and "Once upon a time" are types of commencements in origin myths that announce this. They often then go on to explain how such things as land, sea, sky, and humankind came to exist. Often these claim outrageously short periods as in Genesis where six days of creation are followed by a seventh day of rest. However, just as often, they call attention to a vastness of conception where everything that exists comes into being, lasts a long time, and winks out of existence only to come into being again in an endless round of reshuffling – eons beyond our capacity to fully imagine. It could be argued that the myth – in its poetic expansiveness – is meant to stretch the imaginative capacity of its adherents while reifying its beliefs. But these seemingly exaggerated explanations of origins, if taken literally, have led, in our era that revers science and statistics, to regard these myths as obvious falsehoods rather than poetic creations that explain by propagating analogy.

For instance, the yogis of legend, hidden in the Himalayas, have practices that enable them to do extraordinary feats to defy *time* (living for hundreds of years) and *space* (able to transport themselves astrally). To the *hātha* yogi, health equates with virtue and, in opposition to the restraints of time, yogis claim that one who is accomplished can overcome death and destroy all sins. The soul can be eternally incarnate in *this* material body. This appears to be contrary to the dualistic idea found in the *Bhagavad Gītā* where bodies are predestined to die, but the soul incarnate lives on and is indestructible. But, today, if these ideas are to be totally replaced with notions of health, fitness, and stress relief, the need for such elaborate and poetic myths is unnecessary.

In yoga mythology, light is frequently used as a metaphor for enlightenment (lit. bringing into the light) and the advancement of knowledge. As a result, darkness has been relegated to its metaphorical antithesis in modern yoga. But this understanding of the relationship between opposites is simplistic when one considers both the processes of cognition and ancient yogic philosophy. From the perspective of cognitive science, one learns categories and meanings through contrast. Things are distinguished by their opposites (what they are not) or by gradations of difference where opposition does not exist. For example, good and evil, up and down, and darkness and light are all understood in opposition and tend to be what Claude Levi-Strauss (1990) termed *binary oppositions* – basic cognitive distinctions that lie at the foundation of human cognition.[15] However, colours are distinguished differently across cultures. This is because they are demarcated by arbitrary and culturally specific features that exist on a continuum since no opposites observationally exist. Some cultures distinguish between green and blue, others do not.[16] It is not that the colors blue and green are perceived identically, but rather that their difference lacks significant meaning. Enlightenment, as a process one works toward may be contrasted with ignorance (symbolically understood as darkness), but this distinction is not black and white (as Levi-Strauss may have suggested). There are an infinite number of stages from total darkness to absolute light.

The history of yoga is far more dangerous and violently transgressive than one would be led to believe from the resolutely upbeat image that the general public has of today's practice. The metaphors used to describe practice and its results are often about the light, the enlightened, the luminescent, the shining, or the radiant. But while light may metaphorically speak to us of blissful clarity, it is certainly worth observing that the darkness of such natural phenomena as solar eclipses immediately connect us viscerally with an appreciation of the transcendent. Darkness may prove to have more mythic resonance in yoga in the future. The cultural commentator, Nina Edwards observes, " . . . darkness confers a quality of seriousness, one of getting back to the most basic and powerful of natural phenomena . . . darkness retains this primal gravitas, often becoming a stimulus to religious and other supernatural experience" (Edwards 2018, 56). Acts of profound concentration are often performed with eyes shut creating a deliberate darkness by eliminating the distraction of external light. And sometimes, in this darkness, the other senses become heightened, and things are revealed to us that might have gone unnoticed had the glare of light allowed vision to take its accustomed place of primacy amongst the senses.

The implications for this in yoga practice are important. The ancient yogis believed that darkness was part of the continuum of light, as they both make up the same reality – a light that can be found through the application of yogic techniques. Therefore, they (the 'left-handed Tantrics' in particular) sometimes engaged in "dark" practices – living at cremation grounds, violating food taboos, wandering outside of family and social strictures, and defying even the cosmic order by ignoring caste distinctions.[17] They engaged in these practices to demonstrate through disciplined action that all things are one – that as Ramanuja is said to have stated, the Brahmin priest and the dog eater (outcast) are one in the same. This practice of enacting a taboo to understand sanctioned behavior (through its violation) is common across cultures. In 'rituals of reversal', social rules are violated in circumscribed contexts, inverting the norms of society. For example, on Halloween in the United States, children are allowed to dress up as demons, roam the streets alone in the dark, go to strangers' houses, demand candy from them, and then eat as much as they like. If they are not happy with the generosity of a neighbour, they can vandalise their home. This is an obvious inversion of the lessons taught to children every other day of the year, and it serves to both affirm the value of these norms (it would be ridiculous and dangerous for children to behave like this) and challenge the nuanced aspects of our representations of good and evil. The ritual serves to reveal these nuances through the exploration of what is *wrong* to better understand what is *right*, and is one path for social, moral, and cultural evolution. But, in yoga, whether it is an hour-long class, a weekend retreat, or a month-long teacher training, the emphasis is on articulating and practising what yoga already stands for rather than exploring how those values are established or reaffirmed by their antithesis.

Modern yoga, having simplified the conception of reality to distinguish between positive and negative actions and experiences (possibly influenced by Judeo-Christian doctrine), has relegated darkness to the dumpster along with "negative" emotions (see "Anger Is an Energy", this volume, Chapter 2). If enlightenment is to be defined as an understanding of the nature of reality, yogis seeking it would be remiss to ignore the negative aspects of that reality. Metaphors are powerful, but like binary oppositions, when applied without thoughtful analysis of their symbolic, rather than literal meaning, risk simplifying the understanding of any phenomenon.

Given the eccentric practices of the past, it may be that yoga has transgressively sought to normalise its practice in the eyes of the general public and to align with our modern lifestyle. The back cover of Godfrey Devereux's book *Hatha Yoga: Breath by Breath*, for instance, attempts to clearly state that it requires no adherence to a number of strange customs that might seem transgressive to the modern practising householder.

> Hatha Yoga is not a religion.
> It is not a physical fitness system.
> It is not a stress management technique.
> It is not a cult. It requires no strange beliefs.
> It demands no blind faith.

> There is no need for penance, confession, humiliation, or self-denial.
> It is not a way of life with a special set of values and conventions.
> You do not need to give up onions or meat,
> burn incense, or wear prayer beads.
> Hatha Yoga is more like a science and an art combined.
> There is rigor and objectivity in its method.
> There is beauty and inspiration in its expression.
>
> (Devereux 2001, back cover)

Arguably, the pendulum may swing back to allow for more misbehaving and rule breaking in the service of radical change. What form this might take is difficult to predict. In the 1960s, yoga was seen as a more radical practice sometimes involving the exploration of cosmic consciousness and was associated with psychedelics, communal living, free love, and vegetarianism. Today, many of these practices have become mainstream. However, there has been some experimentation with practices that could be considered transgressive. The renewed interest in psychedelic (ayahuasca, psylocibin, LSD) medical treatment and the legalisation of cannabis have offered opportunities for experimentation beyond social norms. Some have also experimented with nudity as a way to radically break free from norms of both sexuality and decency. But transgressive behaviour is not the same as the deliberate questioning of norms found in structured rituals of reversal. It is difficult to imagine what a structured, periodic, and deliberate practice that is designed to also question, rather than simply affirm yogic practice or values might look like, and whether such rituals even occurred in the past. A ritual of reversal occurs when the social order is deliberately reversed; the world becomes unsettled and then reverts back to order. These rites are important in human culture because they remind us why we have social conventions and rules in the first place and provide an opportunity to evaluate these rules. Many ancient practices were already extreme transgressions from social norms, so it may be that reversal was unnecessary. But now that yoga has been domesticated (made to fit into our normative lifestyle) wouldn't such rituals be useful? The process of creating a ritual of reversal requires that one articulate their beliefs so that these may be violated. These beliefs are upheld and sustained through myth and metaphor which commonly lie beyond our awareness unless there are formalised techniques to reveal them. But these foundational premises are not generally being examined in yoga despite the presence of a formal, ritualised practice structure.

Because contemporary yoga has been denuded of most of the larger questions about the unknown, and domesticated to make it palatable to Western sensibilities, it may be that currently there is no need for modern myths. Just because there are things which are unknown or unexplained, does not mean that they require mythic explanation. For some, there is no need to know a reason; exploration is more important than explaining through myth. Yoga may not have powerful myths today because urgent questions concern more concrete and observable realities like the lack of social justice, the mistreatment of animals, or environmental degradation – for an understanding of these, metaphor may suffice.

## NOTES

1. The *Vibhūti Pāda* (book three of the *Yoga Sūtras of Patāñjali*) tells of the many supernatural powers acquired through practice and the danger of being seduced by these same powers (Satchitananda 2012).
2. The senses deliver signals to the brain and then the mind forms a simulacrum which it interprets as reality.
3. The *Kali Yuga* refers to the era in which we are currently thought to reside. It is characterised by "darkness" or ignorance that cannot be overcome. Therefore, modern practitioners can only have a debased understanding of themselves and reality when compared to the ancients who lived in a time of knowing.
4. In 1893, Swami Vivekananda presented at the Chicago Parliament of Religions and formally introduced Hinduism to the West. He advocated for religious tolerance and the universality of religious precepts. In making his case, Vivekananda emphasised the philosophical aspects of yoga (as a religion) and framed the physical practice of the *Haṭha* yogis as a degradation of the Classical Yoga of Patanjali, (*Rājā Yoga*) outlined in *The Yoga Sūtras.*
5. Languages that no longer have speakers are known as "dead languages". They may still be used for ritual purposes, but absent a group of living speakers will cease to change. Latin is an example of such a ritual language. Hebrew was dead but has been revitalised by the nation of Israel.
6. The *Yoga Sūtras of Patāñjali* articulates the principles of Sāṃkhya philosophy and presents a vision of nature that consists of two categories of reality. *Prakṛti* describes the material world and its nature is wholly transitory. This reality is experienced sensually. *Puruṣa* is unchanging, eternal, and indestructible. This is described as "pure consciousness" and is not experienced sensually.
7. Bikram is known for repeating this story whenever there is the opportunity.
8. Ramanuja was a 12th century Vaisnava sage and Vendantacharya. Iyengar is a caste appellation from the 16th century. It has been claimed that BKS Iyengar was a direct descendent of Ramanuja, securing his lineal descent.
9. The tantric text *Haṭha Yoga Pradīpikā* (15th century) and *Jogapradīpikā* (18th century) are examples.
10. In the *Yoga Mala,* Pattabhi Jois describes the loss of vital energies that accompanies excessive sweating and says that one should only sweat lightly, and this sweat should be rubbed back into the body to restore one's vitality (Jois 2010).
11. *Saṃsāra* describes the constant cycle of rebirth due to the effects of *kārma.* The goal of liberation or *mukti* is to abandon the wheel and merge with the Other. *Mukti* releases us from the suffering which is life.
12. Yin Yoga is based on the principles of Chinese medicine and is much more than the enactment of surrender. It aims to clear blockages within energetic channels and create more supple joints in an effort to achieve a meditative

state. See: Paul Grilley (2012), Restorative Yoga is variable in practice – in the Iyengar tradition, restorative practice is more rigorous in its attempts to gain, rather than release, *prāṇa* through effort. Other forms of restorative yoga, like *yoga nidrā* (yogic sleep) emphasise "restfulness".

13. The imagining of "yoga as medicine" fits within the metaphorical framework of science that is so highly productive in Western culture and central to establishing efficacy in the Western worldview. An entire section at the end of Iyengar's iconic *Light on Yoga* is devoted to prescriptions for healing from a variety of disorders through practice.
14. On one advertisement for the Rubik's Cube, it was said to have "over 3 billion combinations but only one solution" - though technically not wrong, it's quite the understatement, since the number is actually over 43 quintillion (that's over a billion times bigger). However, the phrase "over three billion combinations" is enough to make the point about the challenge of solving a Rubik's Cube, and really this is a classic example of human innumeracy (Pointless Large Number Stuff).
15. In his book *The Raw and the Cooked,* Levi-Strauss goes further to discuss how binary pairs, particularly binary opposites, form the basic structure of all human cultures, all human ways of thought, and all human signifying systems. They are at the foundation of metaphorical analysis and are subject to reductionism as they become mythic in stature.
16. A particularly interesting example is the Himba people, an indigenous population of Northern Namibia. They do not have a separate word to distinguish blue from green.
17. See the various writings of Gordon David White for detailed accounts of traditional yogis and the fear they often inspired.

## REFERENCES

Campbell, Joseph. 2003. *Myths Of Light: Eastern Metaphors of the Eternal.* Copyright Joseph Campbell Foundation, edited and with a foreword by David Kudler, Novato, CA: New World Library.

Campbell, Joseph and Bill Moyers. 1991. *Power of Myth.* New York: Bantam Doubleday Dell Publishing Group.

Cervantes Saavedra, Miguel de. 1867. *Wit and Wisdom of Don Quixote.* New York: D. Appleton & Co.

Devereux, Godfrey. 2001. *Hatha Yoga: Breath by Breath.* London: Thorsons.

Durkheim, Emile. 1964. *The Division of Labour in Society.* New York: Free Press. Second edition.

Edwards, Nina. 2018. *Darkness.* London: Reaktion Books.

Grilley, Paul. 2012. *Yin Yoga: Principles and Practice, 10th Anniversary Edition.* Ashland Oregon: White Cloud Press. Tenth edition.

Holleman, Dona. 1999. *Dancing the Body of Light: The Future of Yoga.* The Netherlands: Pegasus Enterprises.

Iyengar, BKS. 1979. *Light on Yoga* New York: Schocken. Revised edition.

Iyengar, BKS. 2009. "Interview", with Kate Churchill, director. *Enlighten Up* (Balcony Releasing).

Johnson, WJ, trans.1994. *The Bhagavad Gita.* Oxford: Oxford University Press.

Jois, Pattabhi. 2010. *Yoga Mala.* Berkeley: North Point Press. Second edition.

Levi-Strauss, Claude. 1990. *The Raw and the Cooked.* Chicago: University of Chicago Press.

*Online Sanskrit Dictionary.* Accessed 25 December 2022. https://www.learnsanskrit.cc/translate?search=yoga&dir=se.

Oring, Elliott. 1986. "Folk Narratives". In *Folk Groups and Folklore Genres: An Introduction,* edited by Elliott Oring. Colorado: Utah State University Press.

"Pointless Large Number Stuff – PGLN2: Pointless Gigantic List of Numbers – Part 2 (1,000,000 ~ 10^10^10^6). Accessed 19 March 2023. (https://sites.google.com/site/pointlesslargenumberstuff/home/l/pgln2)

Satchitananda, Sri Swami. 2012. *The Yoga Sutras of Patanjali.* Yogaville, VA: Integral Yoga Publications; Revised edition.

Singleton, Mark. 2010. *Yoga Body: The Origins of Modern Posture Practice.* Oxford: Oxford University Press.

Sinh, Panchaqm, trans. 1996. *The Hatha Yoga Pradipika.* New Dehli: Munshiram Manoharlal Publishers Pvt. Ltd. Fifth edition.

Sinha, Phulgenda. 1990. *The Gita as it Was: Rediscovering the Original Bhagavad Gita.* Lasalle, IL: Open Court.

Vasu, Rai Bahadur Srisa Chandra, trans. 1996. *The Siva Samhita.* New Dehli: Munshiram Manoharlal Publishers Pvt. Ltd..

*Chapter* 9

# The Future of Technique

## A PRISON OF ONE'S MAKING

Yoga has evolved in the West along with a system of institutions and prescribed rules for physical practice. As with all institutions, the yoga variety seeks to establish and maintain power over competing institutions and the people who adhere to their strictures. In Marcelo Hoffman's essay "Disciplinary Power" he provides an overview of sociologist Michel Foucault's disciplinary model, as "produc[ing] an organic individuality by exerting control over bodily activities" (Hoffman 2011, 29). In *Disciplinary Power*, Foucault defines members of institutions as "bodies", wherein they are subjected to the modalities of power and become part of the disciplinary system. Ideally, institutions with hierarchal power desire "docile bodies" – bodies that do what they are told in as expedient a manner as possible. Hoffman argues that the body is subjected:

> . . . first, through division of time into distinct segments, such as periods of practice or training; second, through the organization of these segments into a plan proceeding from the simplest elements, such as the positioning of the fingers in military exercise; third, through the ascription of an end to these segments in the form of an exam, and, finally, through the production of a series that assigns exercises to each individual.
>
> (Hoffman 2011, 31)

For yoga institutions, the claimed stakes are high; either follow these practices or, at best, continue to lead a mediocre life (not one's "best life"), or ultimately fail to "cheat death" and be reincarnated into continued suffering. The more astounding the claims made for yoga's benefits within

DOI: 10.4324/9781003471752-13

the yoga community, the greater the justification for this surveillance and motivation for this self-policing. The community – whether it be that found in each studio, system of practice, organisation, or even the worldwide yoga community, has become Foucault's 'panopticon' of sorts. Classical panopticism[1] breaks down what differentiates people from those around them to make them more easily molded and made to fit a specific image that is most beneficial to the reigning hierarchic power. The senior teachers and assistants to *gurus* and celebrity teachers become both the champions and enforcers of this discipline. They themselves are fervent believers in the necessity for policing and the rules and practices in the system and the community itself. Practitioners of set series do not innovate or alter the sequences for fear of being ostracised or impeding their own progress. Panopticism both begs the question, while simultaneously hopes to keep us from questioning, "What individuates this individual?" (Schmelzer 1993, 127–136). It wields meticulous control over the network of power relations that produce and sustain the claims of an institution by means of surveillance.

The thematic and mythic constructs within yoga – all is one, everything is of the same matter, differences are an illusion – also support the erasure of individual difference and have the potential to make group identification and the sharing of yogic values more pronounced. The belief that yoga practice also offers dedicated and disciplined practitioners greater intuition, and through this, access to secret knowledge, also acts as a tool of self-discipline and supports the creation and maintenance of the docile bodies needed to strengthen the community and its leaders.

## Props, Mats, and Other Restrictions

The mats and other props designed originally by BKS Iyengar for his system have become ubiquitous in studios and other practice spaces. These props serve to influence the method of practice and put emphasis on certain aspects of practice. Alignment and a standardised canon of postures deriving from a narrow range of yogic practices have set the standard for "what is yoga", and limited expressions which fall outside of this definition. The mat itself circumscribes the space for each individual practitioner as both limiting and liminal. Practitioners understand the necessity for staying in their space and the violation that ensues when the boundaries of their mat are breached. In a group setting, practitioners are rarely shy about asserting these boundaries, both for themselves and others. This is not simply an act of territoriality; it is an enforcement of discipline and a warning of the potential for reprimand. The ultimate punishment, if one refuses to conform, is banishment from the community. So successful is the panopticon of community that many members will continue to support a system even when its strictures are proven false, or its leaders are disgraced.

Finally, the fact that bodies are the principal instrument for, and subject of, a physical yoga practice makes yoga particularly effective as a policing institution. For Hoffman (and Foucault) bodies (not people, or ideas, or actions) are the focus of surveillance – and they necessarily must be controlled if not "docile" (Hoffman 2011). This is accomplished through establishing distinct periods of training which afford levels of status and, therefore, degrees of both community membership and power within these communities to those that comply – 200 and 300-hour Yoga Alliance recognised trainings, or internal certifying systems with orthodoxies, like those found in Bikram, Iyengar, and Ashtanga Vinyasa. It may establish practice requirements: for example, in Ashtanga Vinyasa one must practice every day except "moon days" (full moon and new moon) when practice is prohibited.[2] Failure to follow these practice requirements will, it is believed, result in injury and the failure to progress. It is also indicative of the lack of dedication that the practitioner has to the institution. Seemingly random details of physical alignment and comportment are given special (if not undue) importance and are universally demanded of everyone (because all people are viewed as the same). Examples include: the heels need to be down, the fingers are all together, the knees must be locked. These rules are applied absent any critical reason (e.g., "*Guruji* says it is so") or explained through tautology (e.g., you turn the hips way out here because it is a lateral posture). Practitioners are periodically tested to measure their ascription to community strictures and their mastery of the discipline required of their bodies. They will gain or lose power within their community based on the results of this testing.

## WHERE WE ARE NOW

Innovation, which has enriched the research and development of yoga over the millennia, becomes difficult if one accepts the "truth" of yoga's modern strictures without critique. In modern yoga, the eight limbs of so-called "classical yoga" have been accepted as the standard for practice and are generally perceived as individual entities that are performed separately. For instance, Pattabhi Jois and BKS Iyengar taught *prāṇāyāma* apart from *āsana* and only to more advanced students. *Pratyāhāra* (sense manipulation) is only superficially taught in the physical practice of yoga. Meditation (*dhāraṇā* and *dhyāna*) is also often a separate seated practice. People often associate the techniques of yoga with the development of flexibility and extreme instances are valorised. Considering how comparatively easy it is to develop one's flexibility, one wonders why modern yoga devotes so many of its techniques to it. This is especially so as flexibility is not particularly advantageous unless combined with a degree of strength to integrate it in one's efforts to find stability or balance (or even harmony in the different parts of the body – making them "one"). In any case, development of flexibility or strength is a simplification of yogic aims. It is fairly easy to improve these outside of yoga practice and it is accessible to most practitioners who desire to work toward these goals. Though flexibility and strength are necessary elements in physical practice, if the *Yoga Sūtras of Patāñjali* is taken to be the seminal text people proclaim it to be, it is the techniques of focus and concentration meant to accompany them that make it a yogic endeavour.[3]

Yogic theory presents complicated models and techniques for bodily processes, as well as for reality itself. Most of these are not testable and, instead, are to be explored by simplified means. For instance, the body might have 72,000 *nādīs*, but only 14 are deemed important and only three of these *really* matter – and two (*iḍā* and *piṅgāla*) have no detectable correlates in a physical body. The remaining one – *suṣumnā* – has some kind of correlation with the spine (Sinh 1997, 4.18).[4] To induce *prāṇa* into this subtle *nādī*, the hydraulics of *prānāyāma* might be used, but because of the extreme subtlety of the structure, the body is not meant to be moved in such a way as to create blockages in this spinally oriented channel. Likewise, models for reality are complicated. *Puruṣa* and *prakriti* are divided into 25 *tattvas* (elements which comprise all matter including mind and action), and there are five major *vāyus* (forces) posited that make up *prana śakti* (the movement that creates in the material world). The techniques in yoga simplify these complex structures (often reducing them to a single element – as with the *suṣumnā,* for instance) to attempt to manipulate them. But these reductions (which offer clarity) come at the expense of experiencing the complexity of a contingent reality. For example, the necessity to keep the *suṣumnā* stable and unblocked has meant that meditation and *prānāyāma* are only practised while in stillness. But one "breathes" when one is moving as well, and the theory suggests that *prāṇa* is always active and, therefore, manipulable. This simplification may result in stifling technical innovation. *Prānāyāma* has become synonymous with breathing exercises rather than principally the manipulation of vital energies.

It is commonly believed that the inhale and the exhale are meant to be of equal length. In *āsana,* this is reasonably easy to maintain. However, with the advent of movement-based yoga – *vinyāsa* – it has become more appropriate and practical to synchronise the breath with the movement; recognising that different movements may require different efforts in breathing. Because the *vinyāsa* philosophy is premised on changeability, the expectation for sameness becomes dubious. No two breaths *are* alike. The best one can do is approximate sameness, but to what end? Comparing with the past, or anticipating the future, lessens involvement in the present. The point of view that the breath should be counted and evenly measured demands the focus conform to some external or artificial order. The virtues of this metered breath are that they allow others in group practice to synchronise their movements and strengthen the mechanics of breathing in a rudimentary way (one technique for learning how to control breathing). This is an example of a philosophy of conformity (as with Foucault's bodily policing) versus a philosophy of unceasing changeability. As a community practice, it raises the question of whether sameness or the appreciation of the uniqueness of each individual within it, is what unifies the group. Metered breath may serve an important and unifying function, but at a certain threshold of accomplishment, practitioners are capable of exploring breathing in a way that is appropriate to their movements. One would assume that breathing is such an integral part of physical yoga practice that it should be taught from the commencement of training. Once the rudiments of breathing are established, the more interesting idea of manipulating energy (*prāṇāyāma*) should take precedence over mechanical repetition.

Classical Yoga has sought to simplify the practice experience by restricting meditative practice to stillness, while other disciplines make movement and meditation fit together. Future technique in yoga could entertain the possibility of integrating the limbs so they become a unified practice. This integration would simultaneously engage more facets of a person's being – intellectual, imaginative, emotional, and sensual attributes – and expand the contexts for meditative experience. The construction of the eight-limb system presumes that there are distinct and progressive stages to yogic practice that culminate in a stage called *sāmadhi*. This separation has led to an atomisation and over-simplification of a complex sensual experience that, at best, provides a description of the processes of meditation, but not the guidebook to the total experience that yoga lore alleges.

## CHANGING OUR POINT OF VIEW

In theory, *pratyāhāra* provides a group of methods that help one to learn to discriminate with the senses. For instance, *dṛṣṭi* is more than where one's eyes are focused. It is an attitude, or a point of view, and may translate to any of the senses. Each sense could be considered when creating a situation amenable to focus and concentration. Focus and concentration are used synonymously, but focus refers to the parameters set around one's attention, whereas concentration is what one does with their intention. Focus is where one chooses to concentrate. Today, the premise of *dṛṣṭi* has also been simplified and diminished. It has changed from meaning "the way in which one *views* things" into "the *thing* that is looked at". In Sanskrit, *dṛṣṭi* can be defined in a variety of ways: vision, attitude, view, opinion, point of view, wrong view, wisdom, theory, system, regard, pupil of the eye, notion, mind's eye, look, intelligence, faculty of seeing, eye, doctrine, consideration, beholding, aspect of the stars, glance, sight, viewing, and seeing (Wisdom Library). The definitions above indicate that *dṛṣṭi* is something that comes from within. However, in Ashtanga Vinyasa, for example, there are nine external *dṛṣṭis*, each designated for a particular posture. One is required to look at the tip of the nose, up at the tip of the fingers, at the middle of the thumb, at the navel, or the tips of the toes (Prax 2019). The subjectivity of the individual practitioner's point of view is forced to conform to the fully delineated form of the posture. The clarity of the shape has become what is important rather than the appreciation of the contingency of reality.

Today it is generally believed that *dṛṣṭi* is performed to create and enhance focus. The underlying premise is, "where your gaze goes your attention goes" (establishing focus), and by looking at a specific point in the external environment, it is thought one can find balance and reduce distractions. The inherent contradiction in the above is that anchoring the focus to an external *dṛṣṭi* is said to improve an inner state (of balance) rather than moving one's attention to the object of focus. Visual focus is perfunctorily addressed in some holding techniques and usually designates body parts as focal points or, if working with eyes shut, an imagined bodily space such as the third eye.[5] Flow practices have been slow to address how the focus is meant to move in the transition between postures and has not attempted to codify the use of external objects. Though there is a general agreement that focus means a limiting of some kind, and possibly an intensification, there has been little critical evaluation. Other movement disciplines have engaged in critical inquiry, experimentation, and formal research on the effects of focus. As a result, runners might focus on the finish line in a race and a dancer 'spots' their turns by establishing a focal point and turning the head so that it re-establishes the focus with each spin. The expansive focus of theatrical performers means that they are aware of the back row of the theatre or performing space. In *Bharatanatyam* (a form of Indian dance), there are 36 different codified *dṛṣṭi* that attempt to account for the portrayal of the range of human sentiment. These practical techniques produce results that may be evaluated and used to advance the discipline: the sprinter wins races, the dancer can execute difficult choreography, and the performer can be seen and heard in a large space. According to David Life, the practice of external *dṛṣṭis* is meant to facilitate the larger yogic aim of looking inwardly to discover the Divine. In a 2021 article in *Yoga Journal*, he writes:

> When we control and direct the focus, first of the eyes and then of the attention, we are using the yogic technique called Drishti . . . Our eyes can only see objects in front of us that reflect the visible spectrum of light, but yogis seek to view an inner reality not normally visible. We become aware of how our brains only let us see what we want to see – a projection of our own limited ideas. Often our opinions, prejudices, and habits prevent us from seeing unity. Drishti is a technique for looking for the Divine everywhere – and thus for seeing correctly the world around us.
>
> (Life 2021)

The connection between limiting the movement of the eyes to a fixed point in the external world is meant to limit distraction and facilitate looking past our "own limited ideas" to see the unity in everything. This justification is given without providing support for how *dṛṣṭi* acts as a technique to "discover the Divine" within and subsequently everywhere (or vice versa). It is unclear whether the discovery of truth comes from an inner knowing (within the self) or is an understanding of the inner essence of the object of focus. It seems to presume that inner distractions are quelled by practicing outer focus and ignores the possibility that whatever is discovered inwardly (whether premised on the "visible spectrum of light" or not) is not generating the same kind of "limited ideas". But does restraint of the sense of vision offer the only method to see the Divine (unity) in everything – or is the expansive nature of looking at a sunset as awe inspiring as limiting your gaze to staring down the tip of your nose? David Life further restates the Ashtanga Vinyasa premise that "[i]n every asana, the prescribed Drishti assists concentration, aids movement, and helps orient the pranic (energetic) body" (Life 2021). This is taken from a *Yoga Journal* article, and not an academic paper, so it is understandable that no explanation is given for how external *dṛṣṭis* assist in either movement or *prānic* orientation. The premise that *dṛṣṭi* aids in movement is simply accepted. Aids to movement are not sought in the meditative practice outlined in the *Yoga Sūtras of Patāñjali* to which the Ashtanga Vinyasa tradition subscribes. To support these claims, experimentation with the manipulation of *dṛṣṭis* could be undertaken to reveal the efficacy of external focal points, the impact of varying the qualities of focus (e.g., intensity, duration, or constancy), and whether inward or outward focus best assists in improving concentration, aiding movement, and the orientation of the energetic body.

In yoga, the aim is often the achievement of a state of peacefulness or equanimity. The ways to achieve this state, however, are defined by what they should *not* be – non-attached, neither liking or disliking, or unmoving.

This exclusion of attributes (and the absence of precise definition) is meant to foster the negation of subjectivity and erase individuality. One is not to be anything. It may assume that the eyes can act as a camera-like recording device – seeing mechanically, without subjectivity. However, even a CCTV camera does have a point of view – its own *dṛṣṭi*. It does not actually record everything – only what is within the limit of its lens and what it is programmed to do. In spite of its advocacy of self-negation, much modern yoga, paradoxically, requires a selective and persistently upbeat point of view (*dṛṣṭi*) – one of compassion, love, and light – that ignores the far more complex nature of reality. It is as though one should aim to be a CCTV camera with a rose-tinted lens. If one is to look at life with compassion, one's point of view must also behold and comprehend its sadness. If one is to experience something with love, this would require seeing its totality – its flaws as well as its admirable traits. Furthermore, the idea of mixed emotions – a sweet sadness or a melancholic love – is not entertained. Instead, yoga technique aims for a fully delineated clarity (e.g., "illusion is only illusion and holds no truth"), that is rarely found in the real world. The information that the senses deliver may be partly illusory, but this does not make their information wholly untrue. The yogic point-of-view, or *dṛṣṭi,* remains unclear because the relationship between yoga practice and its relevance to the outer world is similarly unclear. One would assume, however, that a certain mastery of specific techniques for profound engagement (rather than neutrality or restraint) must occur before one can achieve the state of equanimity desired.

## THE POTENTIAL OF SENSORY EXPERIENCE

The restraint of sensual information is the current method for looking inward, but the techniques of *pratyāhāra* can be much more than its standard definition "sense withdrawal" suggests. Modern techniques range from sitting in a darkened room to lying in a flotation tank to simply shutting the eyes. Short bouts of sensory deprivation have been touted as aids to meditation and relaxation. Longer term exposure may result in confusion and hallucinations. Writers as diverse as Julian Jaynes, Louis Sass, and Iain McGilchrist have drawn attention to:

> . . . the similarities between schizophrenia and the state of mind that is brought about when one makes a conscious effort to distance oneself from one's surroundings, refrain from normal action and interaction with them, suspend one's normal assumptions and feelings about them and subject them to a detached scrutiny . . . The belief that this will result in a deeper apprehension of reality ignores the fact that the nature of the attention we bring to bear on anything alters what we find there. Adopting a stance that

> is normally found only in patients suffering from schizophrenia is not obviously a recipe for finding a higher truth.
>
> (McGilchrist 2019, 333)

The either/or of outside bad/inside good is premised on the belief that the senses cannot provide our mental processes with a completely truthful version of what is not us and this may be regarded as symptomatic of an excessively categoric and rational (as opposed to reasonable) way of pursuing, or thinking about, *pratyāhāric* technique. It fails to account for the possibility that what is discovered inwardly might be just as delusional. The accuracy of both our thought and perceptions are untrustworthy as gauges of truth except in a poetic or metaphoric sense where they can convey the equivocal and sometimes contradictory nature of ourselves and reality. And this is what *pratyāhāra* should help to focus upon. Obviously, working with the eyes shut lessens visual stimuli though that doesn't necessarily mean that the parts of the brain used for processing such input turn off. Traces of light or colour might still be perceived and inner visions summoned up unbidden might appear. However, the lack of visual input may allow other senses to be magnified. This might make it possible to notice sounds (birds singing outside the studio) one had not noticed, and it is also possible to knowingly invent sound. For instance, by pretending to listen to the lowest sound in the room, one's attention becomes focused on an *ekā gratā* (single pointed concentration). How one construes what a low sound actually is becomes an exercise in both imagination and conjuring a vision of reality. In a purely imaginative whim, one might hear a sub-bass rumble and conceive of it as the vibration of the earth's molten core. In so doing, one expands the volume of their consciousness beyond what is physically possible. One danger would be the assumption that this interpretation is real – founded on an objective unchanging actuality – since perception of the universe and of ourselves is always changing. The delight of consciousness is that we can recognise this and adapt to its apparent inconsistencies, adopting ways of viewing it that we can then abandon as we see fit. We are prisoners of this inconsistency and yet, it is also liberating to give vent to imagination.

## Other Senses and Focus

Vision is not the only sense that may be enlisted to establish and enhance focus and concentration. A typical instance of aural *dṛṣṭi* is found when the practitioners listen to their *ujjayi* breath and hear it as the mantra *so'ham.* The sense of hearing has four potential focal points: (1) the sound of one's own body and movement, (2) the sound of the instruction from the teacher, (3) the sounds of the environment which might include music, other people in the room, traffic, lights, and (4) imaginary sounds – hearing the vibration of *Oṃ* permeating all matter around one or listening to the lowest sound in the room or other techniques using imagination. These focal points set parameters around what is intentionally acknowledged and what is excluded to enhance concentration. When the sounds are imaginary, these parameters and the subject of concentration are created within one's own mind yet acted out in the field of reality.

Breathing provides a number of opportunities for *dṛṣṭi*. The act of controlling one's breath creates focus because it requires diligence. Through slowing the breath, the intensity of the focus may be increased. The control required to make the sound (and flow) of the breath even, entails an evenness of mind. The percussive sound of *bhastrikā* or *kapālabhāti* might promote a different frame of mind or *dṛṣṭi*. Because there is a reciprocal interaction between the senses and the thing that they are attending to, smooth breathing and percussive breathing will have different impacts on focus and concentration.

Music and *māntra* are traditional methods for creating focus through attention to sound. Silence is also useful as the contrast between silence and sound may be a point of focus. *Māntra* is no different from breathing in that it is, at one level, a vocalisation of the breath. It is claimed that *māntra* is more profound when executed in a way that is "unstruck", or silently vocalised, because it works on a more subtle level of reality. It might also be that an imaginary act is more perfectly rendered and, therefore, creates greater focus and concentration. The discussion above has dealt with self-initiated sounds. The use of music for yoga engages the practitioner with external stimuli. Music may either enhance or distract but is no different from any other sensually apprehended stimulus – it is a part of the reality inhabited by the practitioner. Music is evocative. However, there is a difference between recollecting experience through music and responding to music in the moment. In the first instance, one engages in another time (there is a memory evoked through the music). In the latter, one's focus and concentration are engaged in a spontaneous relationship with sound in the present.

## Taste and Smell

The relationship between the senses of taste and smell is revealing of the complexity of sensual information. The interplay of taste and smell (and to a degree the sense of touch through texture) gives us what we interpret as flavour. Though the basic structure of taste is made up of only five categories – sweet, sour, salty, bitter, and umami – recent studies of smell intriguingly suggest that humans have the ability to distinguish an astounding one trillion scents (Science 2014). A common example of the interplay between smell and taste is if a strawberry is eaten while the nose is plugged, its sweetness is detected, but it does not taste like a strawberry. It requires the accompanying aroma for the flavour of strawberry to be detected. Similarly, part of the interpretation of chocolate's taste is its texture – the way its fats coat the tongue and other parts of the mouth.

Individuals have clear and strong reactions to odours and tastes. When strong likes or dislikes occur, it is difficult to come up with reasoned responses. Smell is evocative of memories, and as such, can act as a powerful reference or symbol. Incense has an association with ritual and, therefore, is evocative of the sacred and spiritual. This may account for its use in religious ceremonies and in yoga studios. When yoga is performed outside, the smell of the grass, or beach, or forest may invoke feelings of being connected to nature or the larger world.

The utility of smell is various. It is diversely used for such activities as detecting food, sexual partners, and dangerous things like toxic substances. Even minute amounts of scent can activate olfactory memory. That fragrance has psychophysiological affects is clear and this knowledge dates to prehistory. Conclusive study about the nature of these affects is still being undertaken; much of it for commercial reasons. The smell of baking bread may be pumped into supermarkets to influence shoppers' purchases or to entice them to remain longer in the store. This may result in selling more baked goods, but not necessarily other products. By privileging one sensual stimulus over another, the range of experience is narrowed as is the possible effect that may ensue. Also relevant to yoga studios, it has been found that the scent of peppermint affects athlete's arousal, significantly increasing running speed, hand grip strength, and number of push-ups they can do (Raudenbush 2001). Lavender apparently exerts an influence that is calming. Such information might prove useful for developing a sensual atmosphere in a yoga studio, but there are many variables that require exploration before conclusions and viable implementation can happen (Sowndhararajan and Kim 2016).[6] Smell, because of its greater sensitivity and range of interpretation, has vast potential for exploration (perhaps in concert with taste).

Some have already attempted to combine the senses of taste and smell with yoga as a way of exploring awareness. Pairing yoga with chocolate or wine aims to see the utility of yoga techniques in creating or investigating a heightened experience of pleasure. This may function as an easy introduction to focus and concentration because of the ease of gratification. Theoretically, if yoga provides a heightened state of awareness, one should be able to experience taste more fully. But if the technique is being used as an easy introduction to yoga, or a way to enjoy the complexities of wine and chocolate more fully, it falls short of more profound investigation of the power of sensual experience in yogic pursuits. Arguably, one might want to explore unpleasant tastes to see if one can find pleasure (or at least master disgust) in the search for equanimity. By limiting the *dṛṣṭi* to wine or chocolate, one might help to establish a refined focus. But can we establish a broader focus that is more aware of the complexity of sensual experience? *Pratyāhāra* techniques that aim to restrict sensory input could be comparable to the use of props as aids to a fulfilling experience. But is this assisting in advancing one's techniques to achieve heightened awareness, or is it tantamount to what Foucault would see as self-policing? More advanced use of the broad sensory experiences of smell might return to a heightened awareness of the sense of taste and smell in general and what these reveal about the complexity of reality.

As with the complexity of scent, human sight has the ability to distinguish several million different colours and human hearing can detect nearly half a million different tones (Bushdid, et.al. 2014, 1370–1372).[7] The ambience of a room might be conceived as a similarly complex experience as flavour through the combination of lighting effects (sight) and music (sound). Add in room temperature and the smell of incense or a breeze from an open window and it becomes clear that our experience is sensually potent – and also quite manipulable. Our embodied experience of reality can be constructed in delightful ways. The experience of the present, when meaning of experience is sought, reveals it is the understanding that the immediate present is the perfect metaphor for the universal. It is what has been distilled from the Totality into our perception where that meaning is embodied.

## Touch

Touch is so obvious that it easily becomes unnoticed. Physio-taping[8], for example, results in the continuous firing of neurons until they cease to give one the same amount of information about pain. This illustrates how difficult it is to maintain a consistent awareness of physical sensation. Just as we do not notice gravity until it is absent (because it is so familiar and consistent we cease to feel it), touch is hard to maintain because it is always engaged. Given the tactile nature of both *āsana* and *vinyāsa*, it is surprising that more attention is not paid to the sense of touch and the *pratyāhāric* techniques for appreciating tactile sensation and how these impact on focus and concentration. The awareness of touch and how touch interacts with the Other is a central question for physical yoga practice. Practicing yoga in a hot room, for example, privileges one aspect of tactile awareness above others. Substituting outer heat for inner heat may promote a softening or a release in practice, but does heat help or inhibit the effort (*tāpas*) necessary to create it? The stickiness of the mat has become a leveller of sorts – feet and hands do not have to negotiate uneven or slippery terrain as the mat provides an ideal, rather than real, experience of the practice surface and removes the necessity to attend so intensely to touch or accommodate its variability. It mutes the sensations available from the interaction with the practice surface. Sweating is a tangible sign of one's effort in striving and, similarly, the extremity of sensation in an ice bath is meant to induce some psychic state in addition to the sensation. Feelings are themselves a physical sensation and our emotional response is the meaning we give to those sensations. By quelling our emotional responses in search of a state of equanimity, are we withdrawing from the senses? Or is it possible to look for consistency in the way the sensations present themselves in the practice of *vinyāsa* and respond to these sensations (after they are given meaning) rather than react to them?

Touch has been referred to as the "first sense" (Fulkerson 2013) – it is the first of our senses to develop and provides us with the structure upon which we sense our own bodies and first develop our sense of self as distinct from others (individuation). Touch allows us an opportunity for awareness through direct tactile exploration of ourselves and the material world. Touch is so important that losing the sense of touch is often experienced as a loss of self (e.g., the paraplegic who is disoriented because they don't know where their body is in space (Murphy 1987), and touch has such a profound impact that it is not easily forgotten (e.g., the amputee who can still feel their phantom limb).

According to David Linden (2015), there are two main systems of touch: one that accesses tactile information (discriminative touch), and one that generates emotional information (emotional touch). Emotional touch along with interoception (interpretation of internal sensations) is received and interpreted by special receptors which identify touches that increase social bonding (hugging, caressing, assuring) and touches which sense pain, danger, and discomfort (Stromberg 2015). Touch, therefore, plays a role in the discrimination essential for the interpretation of our sense of self and the meaning of our interactions with the Other.

Unlike the other senses, touch is innately multisensory (combines with other senses) and requires a number of exploratory actions to access information and "bind together tactile features" (Fulkerson 2013). To feel for the keys in our briefcase, we employ specific exploratory procedures[9] that detect the coolness of metal, the specific shapes and rough edges, the mobility of the pieces, and the connection of a ring. Through touch one is able to distinguish between a number of tactile features (making it experimentally useful) whereas features are "bonded" to one another when other senses are activated. For example, we can lightly touch an object to know its temperature, run our fingers along its surface to feel its texture, or hold it in our hand to feel its weight. We cannot, however, separate the color of the object from that object as we visually observe it. The color (and shape and size, etc.) are visually bonded to the object. The way that we engage with something through touch changes the way that we interpret and experience it.

This has interesting implications for the physical practice of yoga, since the way we perform *āsana* or *vinyāsa* (which inherently use the sense of touch) will influence the way we interpret ourselves and our interaction with all that is around us. To perceive something tactilely in ourselves, or in the world, and its available features, we must actively explore it. Our ability to disengage features through touch allows a deeper exploration. As Alva Noë states:

> [Exploration] is an extended period of awareness through which we come to feel the various features of the object. These sorts of awareness involve a high degree of novelty; it is not simply the joining together of distinct experiences but an entirely new awareness generated by the combination of exploratory actions.
>
> (Noë 2004, 164)

This moment by moment novel awareness might, therefore, be accentuated through attention to touch. In addition, the sense of touch is amplified when coupled with vision. When we look at an object during sensory exploration, we can heighten the tactile experience.[10] Where we place our attention (e.g., the right side of the body, the feet pushing into the ground, the expanse of the night's sky, the imaginary point of the *mūla*) will change the experience we have of ourselves and our relationship to the Other during practice. As Noë further notes:

> The process of perceiving, of finding out how things are, is a process of meeting the world; it is an activity of skillful exploration . . . we cannot separate out the perceptual capacities from our actions in the world. The general idea of the enactive view is that perception is essentially active, that it involves the implicit, skillful knowledge of how our sensations change in response to exploratory motor movements.
>
> (Noë cited in Fulkerson 2013, 73)

This explains why when we place our hands on our heart, we may experience a sense of spirituality that would otherwise go unnoticed. When we attend to the placement of each *cakra* while chanting the *bīja māntras* for each, we will more likely feel the vibration in the area of that imagined energy centre. This is how the intangible may be tactilely experienced, although it exists only in our imagination.

When things are believed to be "known", they become so fully delineated that we cease to examine them further. Exploration through sensual perception is what brings the material world to life. This heightened sensitivity is characteristic of embodiment and allows us to experience the world more fully. Attention to the senses in yoga practice, in particular touch, offers a range of experience unavailable to those who distrust ("It's all illusory" or "*māyā*") or dismiss sensory experience because rational introspection is seen as knowledge.

## CHALLENGES TO CONCENTRATION

Studies show heightened concentration happens when there are challenges or difficulties to surmount. If yoga is to be more than merely "Eastern Stretch Exercise" or "New Age Gymnastics", it is important that it recognises both its history and its future as a physical discipline that overtly promotes and enhances the ability to concentrate. Theoretically, the emphasis upon concentration distinguishes physical yoga from many other forms of physical endeavour.[11] The styles of yoga that stress considerable vigour have had difficulty reconciling their extravagant movement with the kind of quietude associated with "proper" yoga's seated and silent meditation/concentration. There are, however, trials of concentration where a challenge is made difficult in order to hone one's ability to maintain focus. Psychologists have long recognised that "[h]igher task difficulty makes people concentrate harder to maintain their desired level of performance. As a result, there is an attenuated processing of the background environment" (Sörqvist and Marsh 2015, 267–272). These trials may include the execution of difficult *āsana*, holding postures for a longer duration (e.g., 15-minute headstand), repetitions (e.g., 108 sun salutes), and variety (e.g., remembering the choreography of complex sequences).

There are also conceptual flaws in the kinds of concentration demanded by seated and silent yoga. The classic term for yoga concentration is *ekā gratā*, usually translated as single pointed concentration. The mind is meant to be fixed upon a single point and is to be held resolutely and motionlessly. It is meant to be unchanging. The choice of the single point as the object of attention is an attempt to reduce the substance of consideration to its most simplified state, a place from which there would be no further dissection or atomisation. This is problematic insofar as it is a state that cannot exist in reality. As a conceptual abstraction it can exist, but as such, it can only then be a representation in the mind. For example, if the object of concentration were the single dot found at the centre of a *yantra*, the assumption is that it will not change. Everything that can change is, therefore, excluded. This is, however, an illusory situation. The actual dot, over time, will fade. Even in the course of a single day, microscopic changes will occur to its outline. If it is being viewed in sunlight, the way it is beheld will alter as the day progresses. It is only in a conceptual framework – where abstraction of a single point exists – that it can be said not to change. There are things that do not change. They exist in the inductive logic of a closed system and produce a certain consistency of truth even if it has no bearing on the real world. This realm of abstraction is the home of the single dot. It is a place where background distractions can be avoided (because they do not exist), and the rationale behind changeless contemplation is an ideal.

However, as a procedure for developing concentration, it works. It is incumbent upon practitioners and teachers to admit that it is a technique that does not lead to perfection; instead, it is a step to hone concentrative ability. There is no single unchanging dot, just as there is no achieving perfection. The complete stilling of the fluctuations of the mind, based on the contemplation of an unchanging singularity is, therefore, equally unachievable, though the practice of concentration allows one to approach this. For the movement-based styles, there is a similar need for a baseline that is equivalent to the stillness of mind or unchangingness of the object of concentration. One obvious candidate is the cultivation of evenness of breath synchronised with evenness of movement. This theoretically would lead to evenness of mind (or could be the result of evenness of mind).

Reality is a place where change does happen and that means that a question needs to be asked about whether the background is a distraction or the thing to concentrate upon. Can one, through concentration, learn to see through apparently changeless objects and into a reality where all is unfolding in a contingent, but mostly reasonable way? Concentration techniques may be developed where the practitioner evolves from the *rational* approach to abstract conceptions and into a *reasonable* approach to contingency.

These two kinds of concentration are distinguished by Goethe as 'rationality' (*verstand*) and 'reason' (*vernunft*). "Reason rejoices in whatever evolves; rationality wants to hold everything still, so that it can utilise it" (von Goethe 1991, 821). Though German philosophers were quite interested in this distinction, they saw use in both kinds of thought (and their intersections). The abstraction of rationality and its ability to deliver unchanging facts (discrete bits of information) supports the way that reason functions because it lays out the facts through which one evaluates the contingencies of reality (the holistic point of view). The yogic problem from this perspective is that narrowed focus "cherry picks" facts from a grander reality – it is not adept at observing the whole of reality. It is the understanding of the distinction between rational and reasonable that is essential. The point is to get good enough at concentration so that you can make the wholeness of reality approach the singularity of abstraction by utilising all of the discrete facts, gathered from sensual information, in their reciprocal relationship with reality.

## COMPLEXITY AND CONTEMPLATION

An object of contemplation can be seen in a macro- or microscopic way. In both, there is a reciprocity between the observer and the observed; they are both altered in this exchange. William Blake writes, "To see a World in a Grain of Sand/ And a Heaven in a Wild Flower/ Hold Infinity in the palm of your hand/ And Eternity in an hour" (Blake 1950). Blake's poem works because of the sensual appeal. We know what a grain of sand looks and feels like; we know how a wildflower smells.

The difference between *dhārana* and *dhyāna* is the difference between explicit and implicit. A single dot is just that (not even two dimensional – a single dimension in its simplicity). But the implicit has more depth – it is contextual and contingent. The presence of the dot within the overlapping triangles of a two-dimensional *yantra*, gives the optical illusion of rising on a pinnacle or being at the bottom of a well of triangles. This illusion is the by-product of the interaction between the observer and what is being perceived. The schematics of classical meditation diagrams refer to cosmological vastness and complexity yet are sometimes as simple as an egg-like stone but still indeterminate. They are simply suggestive; it is the observer that provides the interpretation.

The techniques by which *dhyāna* will be practised in the future are difficult to predict, but they will certainly entail some application of concentration to the assimilation of the complexity of the cosmos – both the very small and very large. Many practitioners do not work the skill of expanding their consciousness because they are not asked to, or they do not desire it.[12] Not everyone seeks to explore the mysterious through the senses or the imagination. The limitations to our sensual awareness (based on our physiology) prevents us from having a lived (embodied) understanding of the vastness of the cosmos. This may be an explanation for the imaginative striving for *siddhis.* If everything is one, then while going through the process of self-realisation, one will meet with and then imagine surpassing the limits of the senses.

Whether one is performing a seated, lying down in *śavāsana*, or moving meditation, interpretation requires a devotion of time. The average duration of a yoga class has shortened. If a similar amount of content and comprehension can be compressed into a shorter timespan along with experiential depth, one wonders why yoga classes were once 2 hours rather than 45 minutes. Most likely, the shorter classes are a response to practitioners' convenience, and their more common desire for exercise, rather than engagement in deep contemplation. There are reasons for a deepening appreciation of sensual observation and the knowledge it brings. It is not that the senses are necessarily the most accurate of instruments, but that they are stimuli for our lived imaginations, producing through our mental processes imagery that is unique to each of us – revealing the Self to ourselves through metaphor.

## AWESTHETICS AND LIBERATION

The role of art (as opposed to popular entertainment) is to bring forth something new – to take something that may have been felt in an inchoate fashion and to give it form. A question that vexes some audiences is "What does it mean?" as if a performance is merely a prettified way of saying something that could be made much more concise and explicit with a few words. Music is more resistant to this question than other art forms – it is sounds, rhythm, and harmonies that can evoke much, but which does not benefit from decoding into plain speech. Dance may be perceived as less so. While most people (and cultures) have some sense of what it is to move in response to music, turning this into art has involved formalising techniques to gain better balance, higher legs, more elevation in jumps, etc. and in many instances the physical trick (ten pirouettes, a triple *tour en l'air*) can become more important than the art it is meant to express. The effort of 'Art Dance' to make music visible in human form or to express the stories of characters in a choreographic language are easily lost when the effort to physically excel becomes paramount. This does not mean that this effort is necessarily separate from expression, but many dancers fail to be convincing actors because that is not demanded. In a sense, yoga is at a similar place. The canon of yoga movements, with their emphasis on extreme flexibility in back bends and hamstrings and the 21st century's fascination with the handstand and forearm balances, may be missing out on how these relate to the spiritual landscape just as a dancer, executing superb pointe work, may be doing so absent the emotional landscape of the character they portray.

Great artists often rebel against the limits of the artistic paradigm of their era to develop it further. Yoga can no longer rest complacently in its recognition that "alignment matters", or that "yoga relieves stress". Every other physical discipline acknowledges these things – it is not what makes the substance of yoga. If yoga is there to help comprehend ourselves and the world, it can do this if it resolutely seeks out that which is concealed or only intuited; bringing into the open the inarticulate aspect of the inner life which cultural convention helps conceal. If yoga is seen to be about equanimity, then fears and desires could be brought into the open, experienced, mastered, and quelled. Technique would be used to take the spirit into physical, imaginative, intellectual, and emotional extremes so that they are understood for what they are and can be brought into service or dispensed with. A more adventurous approach to the senses is not without precedence in yoga; the Tantrics sought sensual extremes as a way to understand the true nature of reality against the social conventions of their time. They were ambitious scientists in their exploration of the possibilities for sensual experience and its reproducible results.

How do we take ourselves to a place where we can, with the whole of our being, meld with the Other? To go beyond current ideas about yoga, it is necessary to find new ways to explore it. Standing on a rectangle and going symmetrically through set series of postures has proved a confining experience rather than a liberating one. Different series and different postures are certainly possible as is the improvement of its choreographic complexity (both in terms of meaning and movement). The physical language of yoga and its ambitions are ripe for an extension of scope. The further evolution of yoga is curtailed by the current acceptance of strictures believed to be the inherited truth of the ancients, though the connection between current beliefs and ancient knowledge is easily shown to be tenuous. There never, for example, was a modern yoga mat, yet nearly every practitioner today works on its sticky surface and within its confines. Likewise, yoga was traditionally a solitary endeavour practiced by hermits. Today, group class is a social experience intended to build community. The certainty of belief that we are following a true and unadulterated path becomes its own "prison", curtailing our imaginative, emotional, intellectual, and physical agency. As Foucault (1995) avers, strongly held values, beliefs, and ideals (the internalised controls) are a greater "policeman" than any laws (formal externalised controls). If we believe something is true, we will follow it; if we believe something is wrong, we probably will not, regardless of its legality. What we ideally seek are experiences of awe, where we come in contact with something beautiful, grand, or especially powerful and meet it not with a fear that diminishes us, but with a sense of wonder and expansiveness. Fear commonly accompanies the experience of awe, but in a way that inspires respect rather than retreat. It is tantalising – there is a desire to explore it carefully, rather than push it away. Examples of this are found with people that are thrill seekers. They attest that fear is a necessary part of the positive experience, for if the skill is mastered, it no longer produces the effect because it lacks risk. There is no contingency – some unpredictability is necessary for ecstatic experience, including awe, because that is the nature of reality.

Awe may be understood as "the feeling of being in the presence of something vast that transcends your understanding of the world" (Keltner

2023). The stimuli (which can be sought intentionally) may be found in novelty (new experiences) or the unexpected, but also in the more mundane and everyday – the kindness of a stranger, an ant carrying a leaf one hundred times its size, or the taste of a perfect peach. According to Dacher Keltner and others, awe requires that we "pay attention". Distraction prevents us from experiencing awe; curiosity and inquisitiveness create opportunities to encounter it. The 'overview effect' is a phenomenon where one has the experience of awe after seeing what is familiar in a dramatically new way.[13] This new perspective can be very close up (as in viewing pond water through a microscope) or very far off (as in viewing the earth from a spaceship).[14] We marvel at the indescribable nature of reality, of which we are a part, rather than being dwarfed by it. This expansion or extension is liberation. It is the way out of the self-imposed prison which certainty brings.

## IMPLICATIONS: THE FUTURE IS NOW

Though yoga alleges *mokṣa* (liberation) to be an aim, it is not entirely clear what that means in a modern setting. The most extreme rendering of how the yogic aspirant achieves freedom would be by "dying" to the life they have known since birth (and possibly in previous lives) and being "reborn" into an existence of pure consciousness and, in so doing, breaking the assumed cycle of reincarnation. But how one recognises this state is unclear and the techniques for achieving it are unproven. The essence of it is that the material world is one of bondage – that every action taken in life serves to bind one to a version of reality that yogic lore deems as illusory because our senses, through which we experience reality, deliver an inaccurate (or, at least, incomplete) version of the world which is further distorted by the interpretations made by our minds whose individual capabilities and conditioning invent only a simulacrum of the actuality. Every action the individual commits in this version of reality, more completely entangles them in its seductive appearance. Only through fierce aesthetic rigours can one overcome this persuasive illusion. One might stand on one leg for six years or hold one's arm aloft until it withers ignoring the pain – ignoring all the sensual input – and dismiss it and so achieve freedom from the dominion of the senses.

However, it could be argued that tying oneself to a belief system that includes reincarnation along with a dismissal of material reality is simply another form of bondage – that stymieing one's engagement with life and the enjoyment of it in the hope that an indemonstrable alternate reality will become manifest is another kind of prison. Modern yoga could make a case for construing the prison of traditional beliefs as the illusion. For a prison to work as punishment, the prisoner has to believe in the prison, so much so that they do not even question whether the door is locked. They accept their bondage and whatever suffering or penance that might imply. The modern yoga aspirant is tacitly asked to accept their unworthiness which may be framed as things like a toxic lifestyle or contaminative interest in materiality and the necessity for the purifying influences of yoga. So, when yoga teaches conformity to a style, or obedience to a *guru*, or insists upon yogic lifestyle choices, it runs the risk of being the prison but considers itself to be the means of liberation. One must then assume that, at some point, liberation would be the understanding that one no longer needs to practice yoga in a certain way, or pay homage to the *guru*, or live life according to restrictions associated with yoga today.

Freedom can be felt in many different ways. If yoga is to explore this idea, the way that *āsana* and *vinyāsa* are done will have to evolve – perhaps this will involve achieving a level of physical mastery that allows the practitioner to relinquish the burden of technique. When the technique is sufficiently integrated, then the yogi may perceive that the cell door has been unlocked all along. But until they had the insight acquired through technique, they were unable to explore beyond their prison. What exactly one is supposed to do with the technical mastery of *āsana* and *vinyāsa* remains but vaguely articulated. Seeking technique is a prison if you don't have something to apply it to. The rationale for learning technique is to have enough facility that you can undertake activities you could not otherwise do.

If the traditional belief in an experience of insensate reality that is unlikely to ever manifest is the prison, then one version of liberation is the relinquishing of such beliefs about the future and living through the senses as best one can – gaining liberation by acknowledging that we are already free and that our senses are our own to use and interpret. With this freedom would come a responsibility to oneself – you can (and inevitably, will) make up your own version of reality. One would create a reality that is plausible, and which is also a reality that one likes – and then recognise that any of these simulacrums of the actual reality are provisional. As a part of the material world, they are subject to inevitable and relentless change, but not less enjoyable or interesting for their transience.

> We understand the expression rational deduction as conformity to the rules of logic, but we cannot speak of a reasonable deduction. On the contrary, we can speak of a reasonable compromise and not of a rational compromise. At times the two terms are applicable but in a different sense: a rational decision can be unreasonable and vice versa . . . The rational corresponds to mathematical reason, for some a reflection of divine reason, which grasps necessary relations . . . [It] imposes its themes on all beings of reason, because it owes nothing to experience or to dialogue, and depends neither

> on education nor on the culture of a milieu or an epoch. The concept of the rational . . . is valid only in a theoretical domain . . . When it is a question of behavior, we qualify as 'rational' behavior in conformity to . . . not allowing oneself to be held or led astray by the emotions or passions. According to Bertrand Russell, the rational man would only be an inhuman monster.
>
> (Perelman 1979)

Binary oppositions are simple and afford clarity in meaning. Notable in yoga is the opposition between the *material* and the *spiritual.* We refer above to the *rational* and the *reasonable.* And it is easy to refer to physical yoga procedures that are *particulate* (e.g., focussing on individual body parts – shoulder blades, hamstrings) and those that are *holistic* (e.g., becoming cosmically conscious). A fourth is the idea of mobility or *process* as is found in *vinyāsa* versus the aim of stasis whereby the whole of reality is seen as an *entity* (or object) that is sought in *āsana.* It may be that these examples are actually referring to one and the same thing – a way of perceiving that is engaged and ever-transforming and another that sees things as remote and unchanging objects. Reality might be analogous to the nature of light – when viewed as a wave it seems like a *process,* but which behaves like a particle (a *thing*) if it is pinned down by specific and detailed observation.

Take the first example – the opposition of materiality and spirit. The general public's perception of yoga seems satisfied with a notion that the body equates with the material and the mind with the spiritual. The tangibility of the body is contrasted with the ephemerality of mental process. Many serious practitioners disparage the body and favour the inward looking and intangible realm of meditative contemplation – they prefer "observing their thoughts" and may go so far as to distinguish this process as different from thinking. They view physical practice as merely a preparation for "doing real yoga". Does real yoga actually mean discovering an unvarying place of observation? Physical detachment allows for a narrowing of focused attention (one can then observe a shoulder blade or hamstring) and, in the same way, might prepare one to narrow their attention when one observes one's thoughts. This detachment is transferred into the way practice is done. It results in an experiencing of the body as a number of interconnected, yet distinct parts – the observation of the body and of thoughts literally objectifies them. They become *things.* Some techniques encourage this particulate, rather than holistic concept of body, through alignment rules and in their methods of approaching meditation.

This objectification is justified because it is associated with the way the rationality of science is practised – a narrowly focussed attention (controls); the knowledge of things that comes from the assembling of discrete parts; and reliance on sequential rational logic are all part of the path to comprehension. Objectification works tremendously well at isolating distinct measures of information, so they become unequivocal, but where the edges are blurred or variable, it is less successful. Heisenberg's Uncertainty Principle illustrates this. Commonly applied to the position and momentum of a particle, the principle states that the more precisely the position is known, the more uncertain the momentum is and vice versa. Precision and clarity in one area come at the expense of something else. This objectifying has proved itself adept at understanding detail and at manipulating the mechanics of the world of phenomena but is less adaptable to things that are ambiguous or interpretable like art – or yoga – which, because they do not have a fully delineated clarity, cannot be objectively fixed and then manipulated, and so are seen as more *spiritual*.

A rational manner of thinking is rule based, mechanical, and internally consistent, but not adaptive (e.g., the heels are always meant to be on the floor in Down Dog). Reasonable thinking, which must accommodate contingency, might conclude that it is unnecessary to follow such a rule for several weeks if it were applied when working with a torn calf muscle. The biggest problem with the rational is that, when accepted unconditionally, it makes it impossible to engage in imaginative and adaptive pursuits. Rationality looks at a painting of a table and sees pigment and canvas. It cannot deal with the evocative or metaphoric because these cannot be controlled in their exact meanings. If rationality does accept a premise, it has to embrace it fully and literally. The reasonable sees that a painting of a table is not a manufactured table in the sense that a carpenter would make a table. Instead, it is an expression of something about 'table-ness' and all the things table might evoke (stability or wonkiness, a base for presenting foodstuffs, etc.). It must consider many equivocal or even contradictory concepts of table in the world at large.

Rationality has an affinity with statistical certainty. Experience, something that has unique and volatile meaning or interpretation, becomes something that can be ranked by anyone as a number between one and five. Rational would assume that if a yoga teacher has 100,000 followers in a social media account, their teaching must be good. Such assumptions are made even if it is reasonably assumed that a large number of such approvals come from bots and can be falsely manipulated in various ways. The reasonable sees that an experience is variable and unique – that averaging it out to a single numeric quantity is a meagre representation of the actuality and is used to make the statistical fact manipulable. The sum of this is that bodies – the material – are something that is manipulable because they follow the rules of the physical world and the experience itself registers as spiritual, holistic, and reasonable.

Instead, the above essay suggests that our bodies, in their sensual capacities, interact with the world and are what makes an experience holistic (and reasonable) and that narrowing one's focus to individual body parts or objectifying one's thoughts is a process of the rational. What if our sensual experiences were approached holistically in their interactions with the Other during practice – the body and the mind and everything contained in our experience taken in all at once? Does this experience – any experience – require an observer? A yoga that is predicated on unvarying alignments because they are analytically correct is not susceptible to understanding reality. Of course, there is a foundational truth to alignment (in all physical disciplines), but it only becomes useful when it is returned from an objectifying process to a lived procedure. Yoga has the potential to reveal much about the material aspect of the mind and the spiritual aspect of the body. The body's ability to deliver information and to explore goes beyond the rule-based procedures of logic which are fixed and unchanging.

The way in which the senses apprehend the world, and the meanings that are created in these interactions, are less formulaic or logical than categoric thinking assembled through logical processes. What is pleasurable to one is anathema to another and these meanings are variable too; times and context will change them. This unpredictability is part of the larger picture of reality where the focus takes in more detail, which may be mutable, and which contains that which conflicts but does not annihilate (e.g., wet and dry exist where the ocean meets the beach – it accepts the relative; the gradation of meaning between absolutes).

The fixity of focus – *ekā gratā* – has largely been interpreted as an exercise in objectification. One direction that yoga may explore in the future is that the volume of its focus is as important as the fixity on a single point. This would create an increased emphasis on process as opposed to stasis. Recognition that consciousness is an intersubjectivity between self and reality could mean that more than lip service is paid to yoga messaging like "the journey is more important than the destination". The point of the senses, however imperfect they may be, is that they are a connection to the Other. They present information to interpret and would undoubtedly be a part of a yoga of engagement as opposed to objectification. Naturally, this engagement entails a commitment to interpretation of some sort, but in a reality where all is change then that commitment is regarded as temporary. Slogans like "Just do it" or "Just try" have found contemporary resonance because they suggest, in an age of *anomie*, that profound engagement is possible and that the word 'just' implies that giving it a go is what makes for satisfying practice and philosophy.

For this to occur, it is necessary for people to enjoy Sontag's "the ecstasy of surrender" (Sontag 1966) with their bodies and the activities they can engage in. The nature of physical practice in yoga has historically been one of restriction and containment because it has been seen as a distraction from the 'Classical' goal of stilling the mind. There is a disciplining of the body to gain control over it – alignment being the final rationale rather than a gateway for exploration. What if a future goal included freeing the body in an effort to liberate the mind?

The most radical departure that yoga could make would be to finally liberate itself from both the past and the future – the final acceptance that when we die, we die. There is no greater meaning to it, there is no transmigrating soul, there is no heaven and no hell, there is no God, and there is no benevolent universe giving us the education we need. Nothing we do makes any difference in the vast scheme of things – it only makes a difference to us. So, we are free to live how we like. It is a freedom that is open to terrible abuse. Each of us would accept responsibility for their beliefs, for their own moral code, and for their aesthetic tastes and such a responsibility most seem ill-equipped to bear. If you did things that made you feel unwell or unhappy, would you keep repeating them? When it comes to doing yoga, presumably, at present, it is something that people do by choice, so it is curious that few are prepared to arduously follow the life of a yogi and, at most, will choose to be a yoga teacher. Most people lack the strength to do what they really wish to do. The actuality is that each of us has a body, and it is employed in negotiating the rest of reality. The way that it does this has been artlessly refined over millions of years, but each individual model has a very limited life span during which there is nothing that *has* to be accomplished except that which we each individually choose. As the chapters in this book suggest, the body is here for us – the function of technique is to use it well.

## NOTES

1. The panopticon is a type of institutional building designed by the English philosopher and social theorist Jeremy Bentham in the 18th century. The design of the panopticon allows all prisoners of an institution to be observed by a single security guard, without the inmates being able to tell whether they are being watched. It is impossible for the single guard to observe all the inmates' cells at once, but because the inmates cannot know when they are being watched, they are motivated to act as though they are always being watched – the inmates are effectively compelled to regulate (police) their own behaviour.
2. Moon Days may be defined as days when there is a full moon or a new moon. Systems like Iyengar also prohibit practice during menses unless it is a "menstrual practice" – a special sequence of postures which is performed in an area away from other practitioners.
3. It seems more likely, therefore, that the emphasis on flexibility is connected to the increasing importance of the execution of extreme postures in highly

prescribed ways. If one is to be able to follow the prescribed alignment for *trikoṇāsana* (triangle pose) in the Iyengar system, for example, one needs to be flexible enough to place their palm flat on the ground outside their ankle. Similarly, one must be able to get both legs wrapped behind their head to advance to the second series in Ashtanga Vinyasa.

4. 4:18 *Haṭha Yoga Pradīpikā* In this body there are 72,000 openings of *nadis*: of these, the *suṣumnā,* which has the *śāmbhavīśakti* in it, is the only important one, the rest are useless.
5. External objects such as candle flames or *yantras* may be used as focal points in meditative practices.
6. The study by Sowndhararajan and Kim, (2016) looks at the effect of many different fragrances on electroencephalographic readings and concludes with this comment. The concentration of the fragrances also plays a major role in EEG activity, because a higher concentration provides a higher fragrance density. Hence, results may differ when using different concentrations of the fragrance. Moreover, the EEG recording time is a very important factor in attaining constant EEG readings from various laboratories. Therefore, it is still unknown whether the fragrances will show the same effect for a longer duration of EEG recordings with different concentrations and more participants. In light of these limitations, standardising and developing a common standard operating procedure for the effect of fragrances on EEG activity (such as recording time, administration method, concentration of fragrance, number of electrode sites and placebo) is necessary. Only then will we be able to understand the exact action of fragrances on human brain function in relation to EEG brain wave changes.
7. According to Bushdid, Magnasco, Vosshall, and Keller (2014), colour stimuli vary in wavelength and intensity. Tones vary in frequency and loudness. Smell, however, doesn't have any known dimensions. This has made it difficult for researchers to pinpoint how many different scents, or olfactory stimuli, we can distinguish. A study from the 1920s suggested that humans could discern about 10,000 smells—a number far below our other senses. Odours almost always represent mixtures of many different components in various ratios. The scent of a rose, for example, is made up of a mix of 275 components, with only a few contributing to the smell we perceive.
8. Taping or strapping is a technique used by physiotherapists for injury prevention or rehabilitation. It helps to reduce pain by stimulating movement detectors in the nerve (mechanoreceptors) which stop messages passing via pain receptors (nociceptors).
9. Exploratory procedures are specialised patterns of tactile exploration linked to specific aspects of objects. They include 'lateral motion' to assess surface texture, 'pressure' to assess hardness, 'static motion' to assess temperature, 'unsupported holding' to assess weight, 'enclosure' to assess volume or global shape, and 'contour following' to assess exact shape.
10. Like touch, vision is exploratory. We scan our environment to pick up the visual cues we need to understand and interact in our environment. Vision like touch, therefore, requires skilfully executed actions.
11. Many physical activities emphasise focus and concentration because they require a level of physical skill to ensure they are safely accomplished, e.g., rock climbing, slack lining, martial arts, etc.
12. Many practitioners see contemplation as a "spiritual" endeavour, and they are just in it for the physical exercise.

13. The overview effect is a cognitive shift reported by some astronauts while viewing the Earth from space. Researchers have characterised the effect as a state of awe with self-transcendent qualities, precipitated by a particularly striking visual stimulus (Vosky 2020).
14. In a sun salute in yoga, you may experience magnification effect if you practice with your eyes closed with a focus on the imaginary third eye as it travels through space. Likewise, you may experience the vastness and your connection to it if in this same sun salute your focus is on the space around you.

## REFERENCES


Blake, William. 1950. "Auguries of Innocence". In *Poets of the English Language*, edited by WH Auden and Norman Holmes Pearson. New York: Viking Press.

Bushdid, C., MO Magnasco, LB Vosshall, and A. Keller. 2014. "Humans Can Discriminate More Than 1 Trillion Olfactory Stimuli". *Science* 343 (6177): 1370–1372.

Foucault, Michel. 1995. *Discipline and Punish: The Birth of the Prison*, translated by Alan Sheridan. New York: Vintage Books. Second edition.

Fulkerson, Matthew. 2013. *The First Sense*. Boston: MIT Press.

von Goethe, Johann Wolfgang. 1991[1833]."Maximen und Reflektionen". In *Samtliche Werke*, vol. 17, edited by K. Richter and Carl Hanser. Munich: Verlag.

Hoffman, Marcelo. 2011. "Disciplinary Power". In *Michel Foucault: Key Concepts*, edited by Dianna Taylor. Durham: Acumen.

Keltner, Dacher. 2023. "How a Bit of Awe Can Improve Your Health". *NYT* 3 January 2023. Accessed 5 February 2023. https://www.nytimes.com/2023/01/03/well/live/awe-wonder-dacher-keltner.html.

Life, David. 2021. "See More Clearly by Practicing Drishti". *Yoga Journal* 1 October 2021, Accessed 29 December 2023. https://www.yogajournal.com/yoga-101/philosophy/the-eye-of-the-beholder/.

Linden, David. 2015. *Touch: The Science of Hand, Heart, and Mind*. London: Penguin.

McGilchrist, Iain. 2019. *The Master and His Emissary*. New Haven and London: Yale University Press.

Murphy, Robert. 1987. *The Body Silent*. New York: Henry Holt & Co.

Noë, Alva. 2004. *Action in Perception*. Cambridge, MA: MIT Press.

Perelman, Chaïm. 1979. *The Rational and The Reasonable*. The New Rhetoric and the Humanities. Synthese Library, vol 140. Dordrecht: Springer. https://doi.org/10.1007/978-94-009-9482-9_11.

Prax, Alina. 2019. "The 9 Drishtis of Ashtanga Yoga". *Yogapedia* 27 December 2019 (Updated: 26 August 2020). Accessed 31May 2023. https://www.yogapedia.com/the-9-drishti-of-yoga/2/9747.

Raudenbush, Bryan, Nathan Corley, and William Eppich. 2001. "Enhancing Athletic Performance Through Administration of Peppermint Odor". *Journal of Sport and Exercise Psychology* 23 (2): 156–160. doi: 10.1123/jsep.23.2.156.

Schmelzer, Mary. 1993. "Panopticism and Postmodern Pedagogy." *Foucault and the Critique of Institutions*, edited by John Caputo and Mark Yount, 127–136. University Park: Pennsylvania State University Press.

*Science*. 2014. 343 (6177): 1370–1372. doi: 10.1126/science.1249168.

Sinh, Pancham. 1997. *The Hatha Yoga Pradipika.* Fifth edition. New Delhi: Munshiram Manoharlal Publishers Pvt. Ltd.

Sontag, Susan. 1996. *Against Interpretation, and Other Essays.* New York: Farrar, Straus & Giroux.

Sörqvist, Patrik and John E. Marsh. 2015. "How Concentration Shields Against Distraction". *Current Directions in Psychological Science* 24 (4): 267–272. doi: 10.1177/0963721415577356. PMID: 26300594; PMCID: PMC4536538.

Sowndhararajan, Kandhasamy and Songmun Kim. 2016. "Influence of Fragrances on Human Psychophysiological Activity: With Special Reference to Human Electroencephalographic Response". *Scientia Pharmaceutica* 84 (4): 724–751. doi: 10.3390/scipharm84040724.

Stromberg, Joseph. 2015. "9 Surprising Facts About the Sense of Touch". *Vox* 29 January 2015. Accessed 3 January 2023. https://www.vox.com/2015/1/28/7925737/touch-facts.

Vosky, Anaïs. 2020. "The Ecological Significance of the Overview Effect: Environmental Attitudes and Behaviours in Astronauts". *Journal of Environmental Psychology* 70: 101454. Accessed 3 February 2023. https://www.sciencedirect.com/science/article/abs/pii/S0272494420300517.

*Wisdom Library.* Accessed 6 January 2023. https://www.wisdomlib.org/definition/drishti.

# Index